최상위 3%를 위한 책

산부인과
FINAL CHECK

병리

PATHOLOGY

최원규 지음

군자출판사

산부인과
FINAL CHECK │ 병리

첫째판 1쇄 인쇄 │ 2022년 5월 9일
첫째판 1쇄 발행 │ 2022년 5월 20일

지 은 이   최원규
발 행 인   장주연
출 판 기 획   최준호
편집디자인   최정미
표지디자인   김재욱
발 행 처   군자출판사(주)
         등록 제 4-139호(1991. 6. 24)
         본사 (10881) **파주출판단지** 경기도 파주시 회동길 338(서패동 474-1)
         전화 (031) 943-1888   팩스 (031) 955-9545
         홈페이지 │ www.koonja.co.kr

ISBN 979-11-5955-891-7
     979-11-5955-888-7 (세트)

정가 50,000원

최상위 3%를 위한 책

산부인과
FINAL CHECK

병리

Contents

산부인과
FINAL CHECK | 병리

산부인과
FINAL CHECK

병리

PATHOLOGY

I. Cervical cytology

01 Trichomonas vaginalis

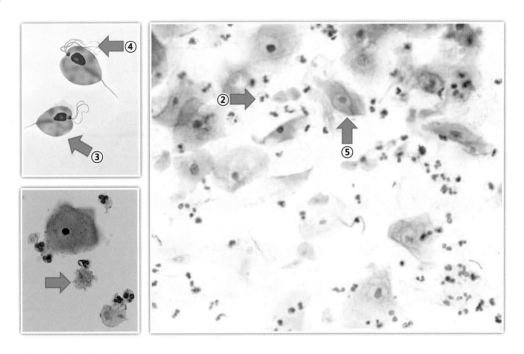

① Pear-shaped, oval to round or kite shaped

② Pale, vesicular and centrally located nuclei

③ Eosinophilic cytoplasmic granules

④ Flagella

⑤ Commonly associated with acute inflammation, lymphocytes, degeneration squamous cells

02 Candida albicans

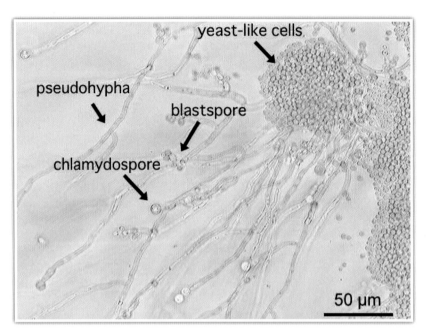

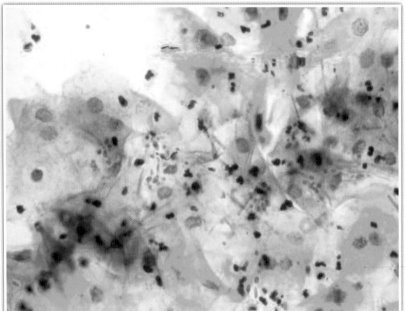

① The budding yeast form and pseudohyphae

② Shish kebab : Reactive squamous epithelial cells in the form

03 Bacterial vaginosis

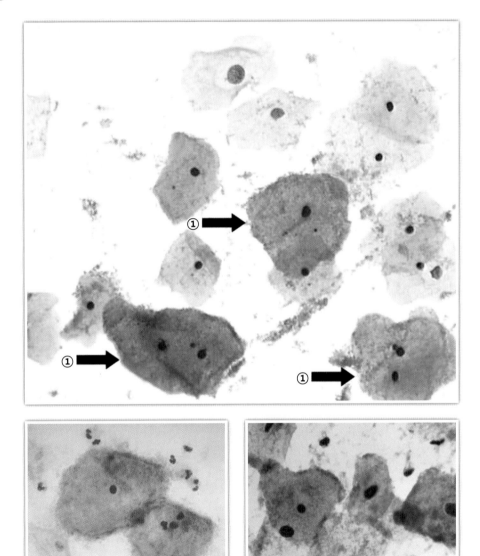

① Clue cells : Squamous cells covered by coccobacilli with extension to the cell edges

② The entire cell does not need to be covered

③ Lactobacilli and inflammatory cells are absent, unless there is another infectious process

④ The small coccobacilli form a granular blue background on conventional smears

04 Actinomycosis

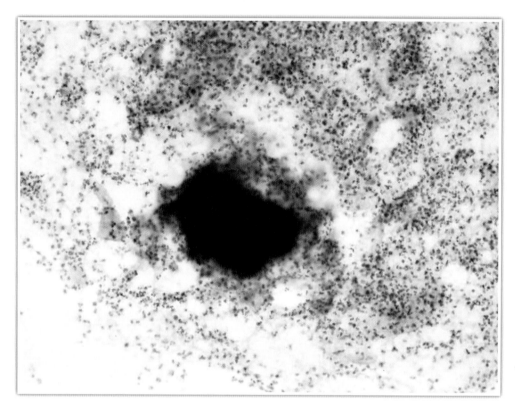

① Aggregates of pseudofilamentous material, often with acute angle branching

② Cotton ball : Tangled clumps of filamentous organisms

05 Lactobacilli

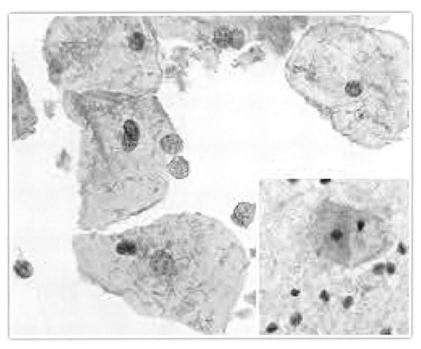

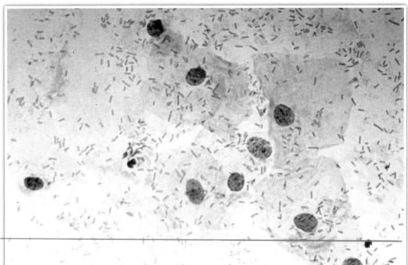

① Bacterial cytolysis : Bare nuclei of intermediate cells and many lactobacilli in the background

② Cytolysis is limited to intermediate cells

③ Cytolysis does not affect dysplastic cells

06 Herpes simplex virus (HSV)

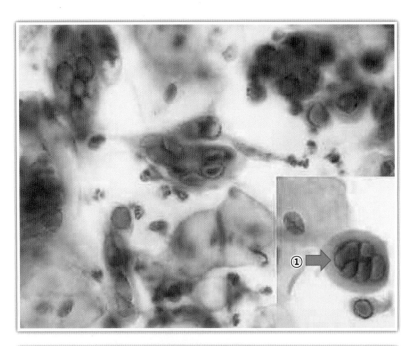

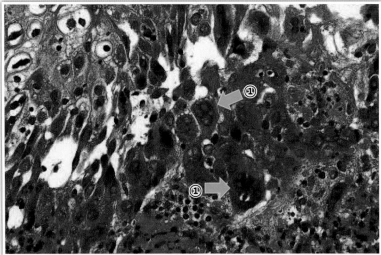

① Multinucleated giant cells with the eosinophilic intranuclear inclusions

② Nuclei have ground glass appearance due to accumulation of viral particles, which causes peripheral margination of chromatin

③ Three M : Margination of nuclei, Molding, Multinucleation

II. Benign glandular tumors and tumor-like lesions

01 Endocervical polyp

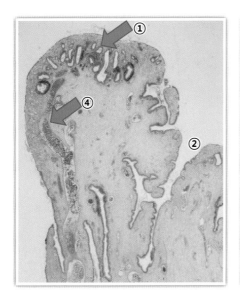 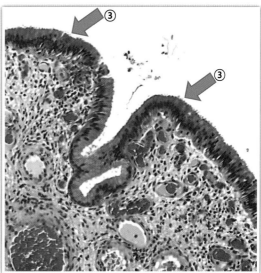

① Dilated endocervical glands in inflamed, myxoid stroma

② Papillary endocervicitis if branching papillary structure

③ Surface epithelium may show squamous metaplasia

④ Thick-walled blood vessels at base of polyp

⑤ No mitotic figures

02 Microglandular hyperplasia

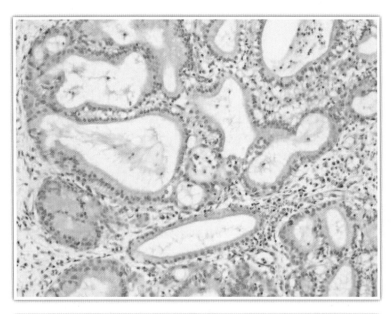

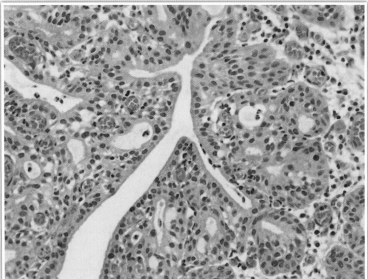

① Complex proliferation of small back to back glands lined by cuboidal, columnar or flattened cells with prominent vacuoles above/below vesicular nuclei

② Indistinct nucleoli, usually no atypia

③ May be associated with immature or mature squamous metaplasia

III. Premalignant squamous lesions

01 HPV infection

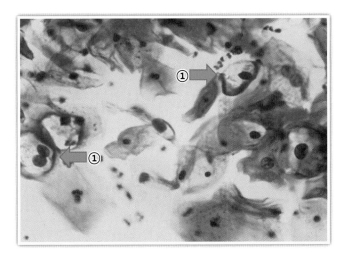

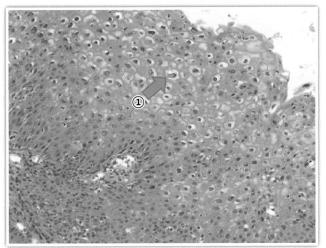

① Koilocytosis

    a. Expression of viral E4 protein and disruption that this causes in cytoplasmic keratin matrix

    b. Perinuclear halo(clear perinuclear zone)

    c. Dense peripheral cytoplasmic rim

    d. Enlarged wrinkled nuclei

② Normal basal cell layer, expanded parabasal cell layer, with orderly maturation

02 Condyloma acuminatum

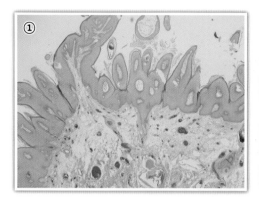

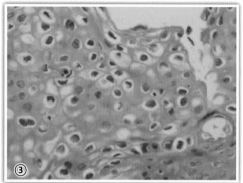

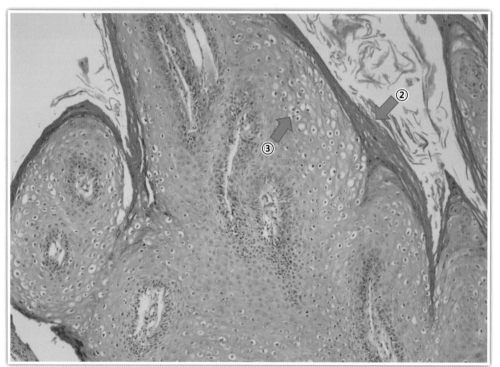

① Verruciform growth pattern with blunt shaped papillae acanthosis

② Hyperkeratosis

③ Koilocytosis

03 자궁경부 편평상피세포암의 전구들에 대한 분류 체계의 비교

Dysplasia/Carcinoma in situ	Cervical Intraepithelial Neoplasia (CIN)	Squamous Intraepithelial Lesion (SIL)
Mild dysplasia	CIN 1	Low-grade SIL (LSIL)
Moderate dysplasia	CIN 2	High-grade SIL (HSIL)
Severe dysplasia	CIN 3	High-grade SIL (HSIL)
Carcinoma in situ	CIN 3	High-grade SIL (HSIL)

Cytology

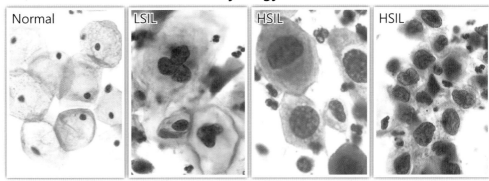

Histology

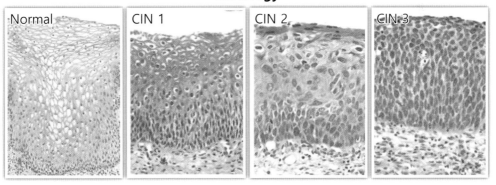

04 LSIL

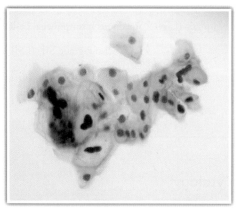
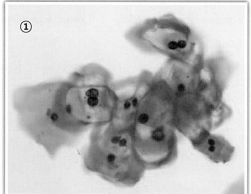

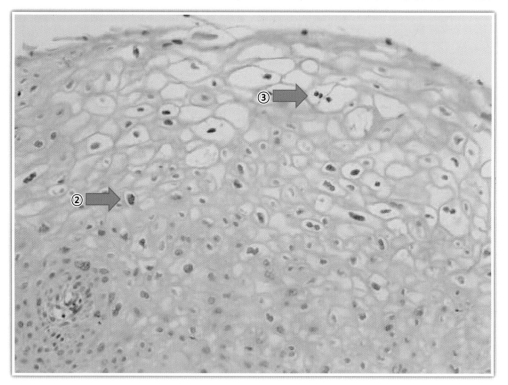

① Koilocytosis : Surface에서만 관찰됨

② N/C ratio 증가 : 중간세포 핵의 3배 이상

③ 핵이 2개 보이기도 함

05 HSIL

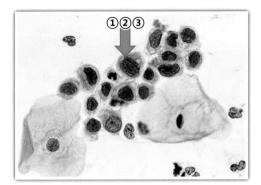 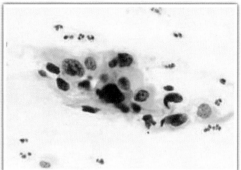

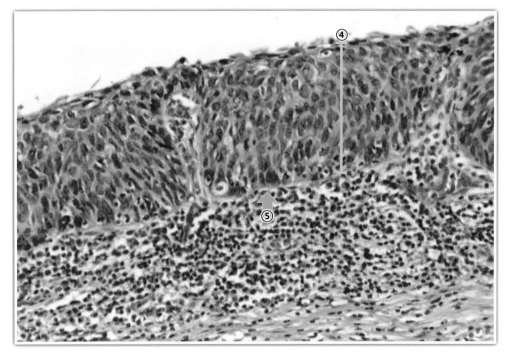

① High N/C ratio

② Wavy nuclear membrane

③ Coarse chromatin

④ CIN 3

   a. 전층에 걸쳐 density가 비슷함

   b. Intact basement membrane

06 Microinvasive squamous cell carcinoma

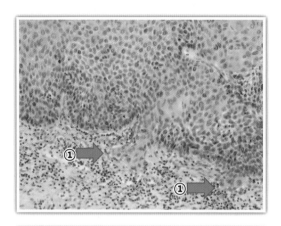

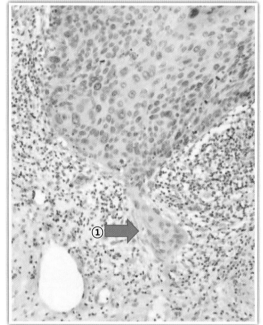

① Irregularly shaped tongues of epithelium projecting into stroma

② Invasive cells exhibit individual cell keratinization, loss of polarity, pleomorphism, cellular differentiation, prominent nucleoli, desmoplastic stroma rich in acid mucosubstances with metachromatic staining properties, breach of basement membrane by reticulin stains

③ Scalloped margins at epithelial-stromal interface, duplication of neoplastic epithelium or pseudoglands

07 Squamous cell carcinoma

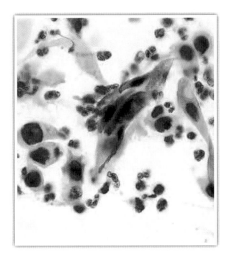

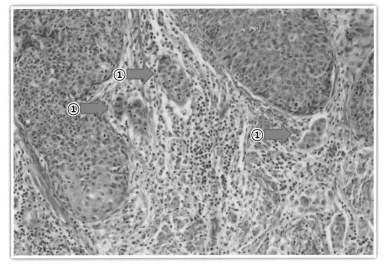

① Invasion characterized by desmoplastic stroma, focal conspicuous maturation of tumor cells with prominent nucleoli, blurred or scalloped epithelial-stromal interface, loss of nuclear polarity

② May have pseudoglandular pattern due to acantholysis and central necrosis

③ May have HSIL/CIN III like growth pattern

08 Squamous cell carcinoma, Keratinizing type

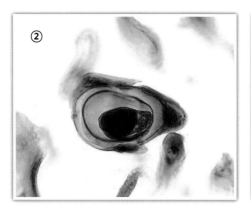
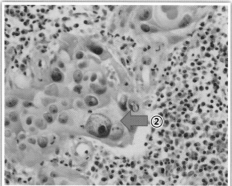

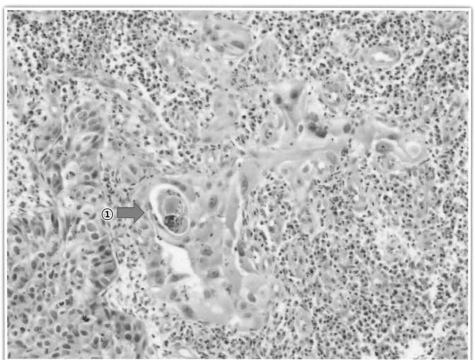

① Must have keratin pearls and intercellular bridges to be keratinizing

② Keratin pearl : Round nest of squamous epithelium with circles of squamous cells surrounding a central focus of acellular keratin

③ Cells are large with abundant eosinophilic cytoplasm

④ Nuclei may be enlarged or pyknotic

09 Squamous cell carcinoma, Non-keratinizing type

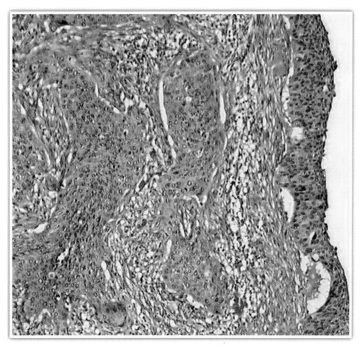

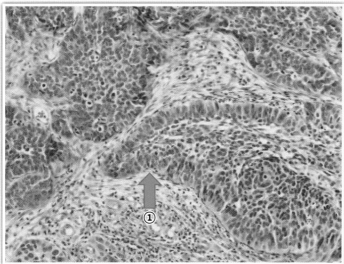

① Rounded nests of neoplastic squamous cells with no keratin pearls, but may have individual cell keratinization or clear cells

② Relatively uniform cells with indistinct cell borders and numerous mitotic figures

IV. Glandular tumors and precursors of the uterine cervix

01 Adenocarcinoma in situ (Endocervical type)

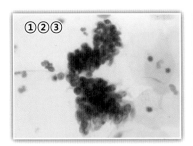 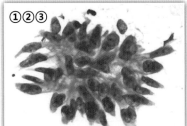

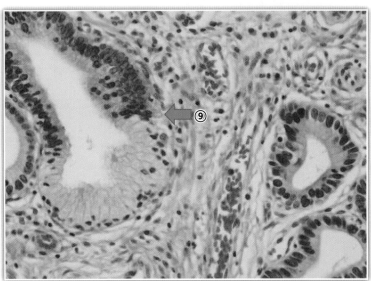

① Nuclear stratification and loss of polarity

② Nuclear atypia and hyperchromasia

③ Macronucleoli

④ Loss of intracytoplasmic mucin

⑤ Increased mitotic activity

⑥ Atypical mitoses

⑦ Apoptotic bodies

⑧ Goblet cells (also neuroendocrine & Paneth cells)

⑨ Abrupt transition to normal

02 Adenocarcinoma in situ (Gastric type)

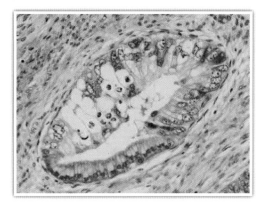

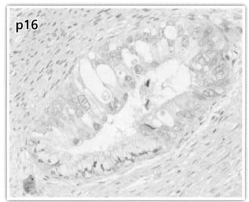

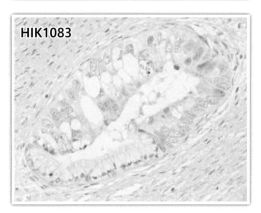

① Endocervical gland lined by tall columnar cells with abundant clear or pale eosinophilic cytoplasm
   and distinct nuclear anaplasia

② p16 : negative, HIK1083 : focal positive

03 Endocervical adenocarcinoma

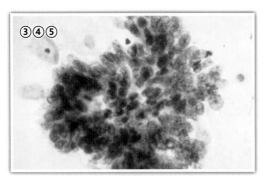

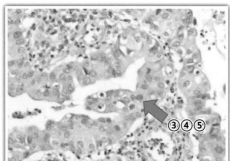

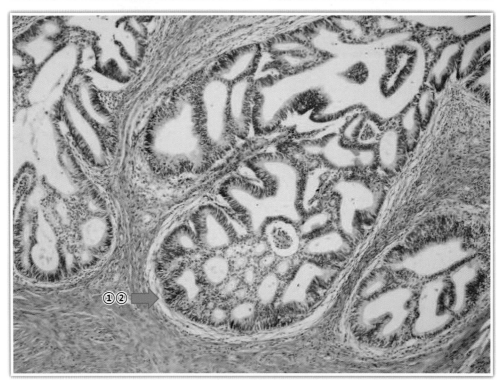

① Cribriform glands : Gland 하나에 여러 개의 lumens

② Irregular shaped gland

③ Peudostratification

④ Prominent nucleoli

⑤ Nuclear crowding

04 Mucinous adenocarcinoma

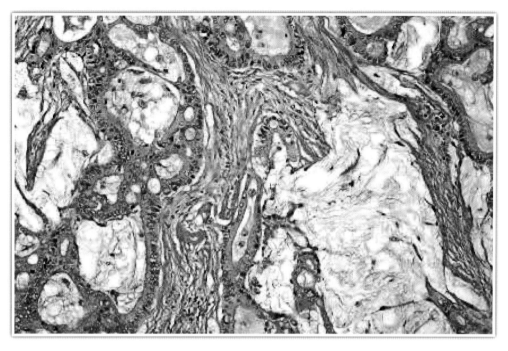

① An invasive adenocarcinoma that shows evidence of mucinous differentiation

② But does not show the specific features of usual type, gastric type, intestinal type or signet ring cell type adenocarcinoma

05 Mucinous adenocarcinoma (Gastric type)

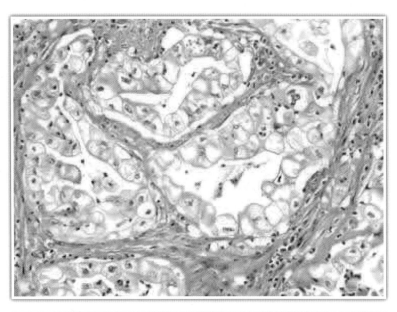

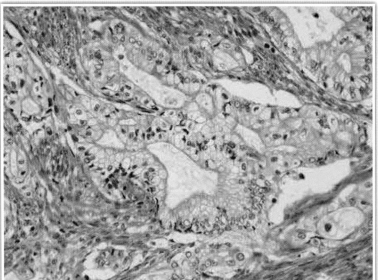

① Atypical nuclei

② Abundant cytoplasm

③ Prominent cell membrane

④ Irregularly fused neoplastic glands

06 Mucinous adenocarcinoma (Intestinal type)

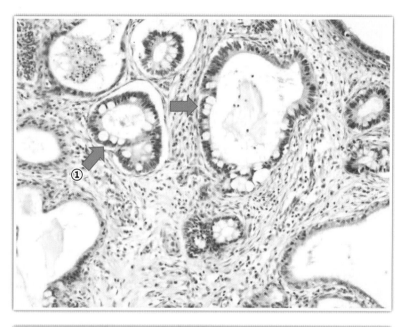

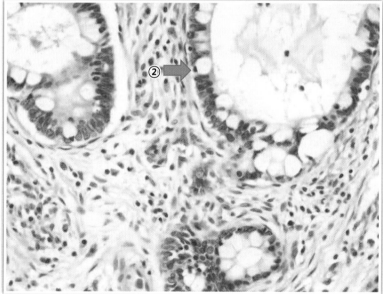

① Mimics colonic epithelium; glands lined by pseudostratified, malignant appearing cells with intra-cytoplasmic mucin vacuoles

② Goblet cells

07 Minimal deviation adenocarcinoma (Adenoma malignum)

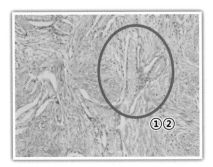

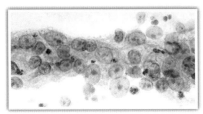

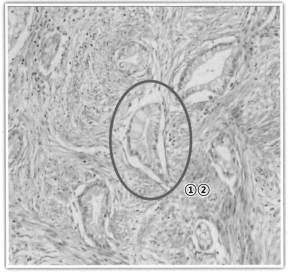

① Very well differentiated glands with cystic dilation

② Glands are variable in shape or size with irregular or claw-shaped outlines

③ Malignant due to distorted glands with irregular outlines deep in cervix, focal stromal response

④ 50% have small foci with a moderate/poorly differentiated focus

08 Mucinous adenocarcinoma (Endometroid type)

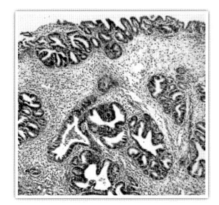
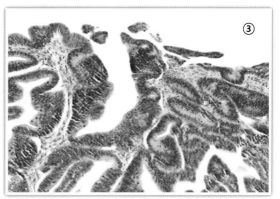

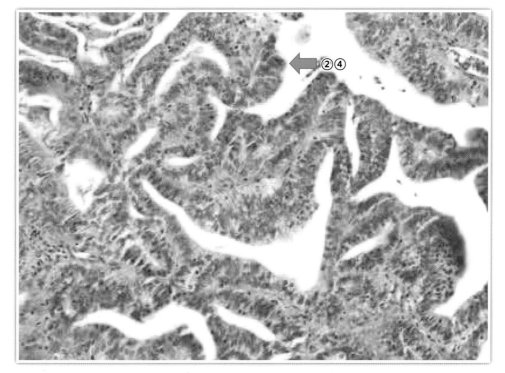

① Resembles tumor in uterine corpus and ovary

② Often well differentiated

③ Complex branching of glands lined by pseudostratified cells with scant cytoplasm and no mucin vacuoles present on H&E

④ Crowded and stratified nuclei

09 Clear cell carcinoma

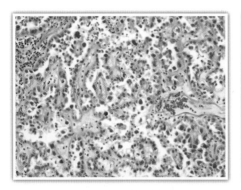
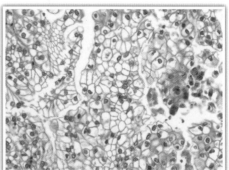

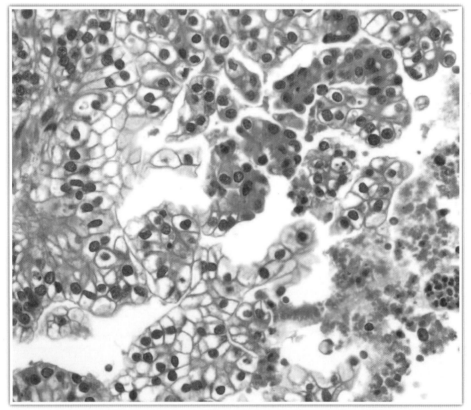

① Tubulocystic, solid, papillary or microcystic patterns of cells with abundant clear or eosinophilic cytoplasm, large irregular nuclei

② Hobnailing of cells : Nuclei protrude into lumina

③ Intraglandular papillary projections

10 Serous papillary carcinoma

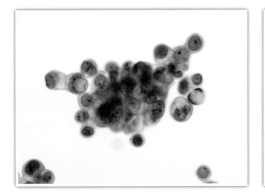
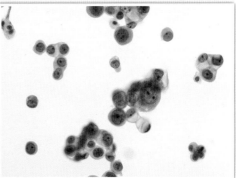
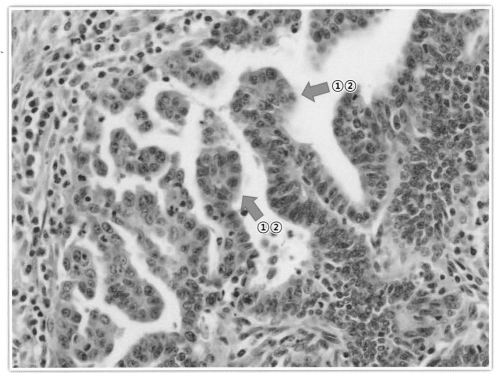

① Papillary proliferation of pleomorphic epithelial cells with complex papillary architecture on fibro-vascular cores, exhibiting epithelial stratification and tufting

② Cells have protruding apical cytoplasm, nuclear atypia and nuclear pleomorphism

③ Mitotic activity, Psammoma bodies : common

I. Cyclic change of endometrium

01 Basalis of the endometrium

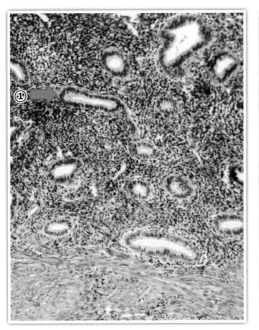 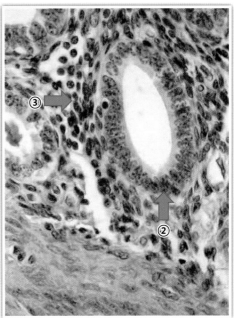

① Inactive gland가 관찰

② Atrophic endometrium 양상의 single layer culumnar cell

③ 사이사이의 stroma

02 Mid-proliferative endometrium

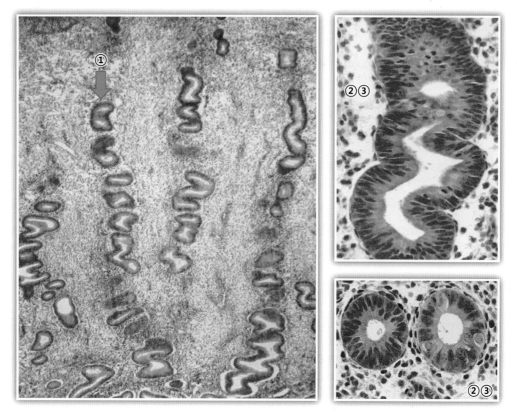

① The early coiling

② Synchronously developed glands

③ Elongated glandular nuclei, pseudostratified

03 Early secretory endometrium

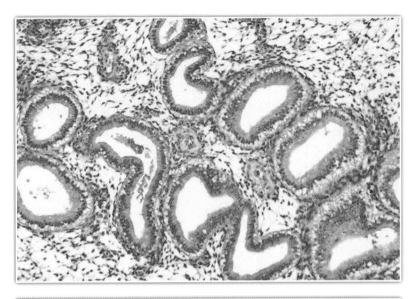

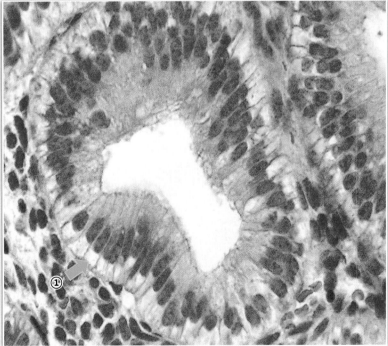

① Subnuclear vacuoles

② 36 hours after ovulation

04 Mid-secretory endometrium

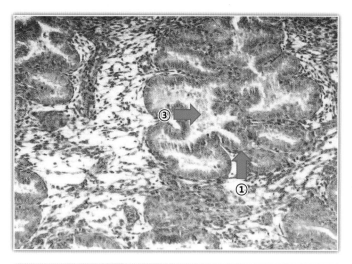

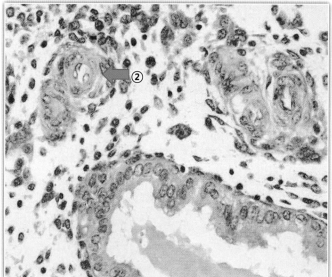

① Extreme glandular coiling & stromal edema

② The coiled spiral arteries within an edematous stroma

③ Intraluminal secretion

05 Late secretory endometrium

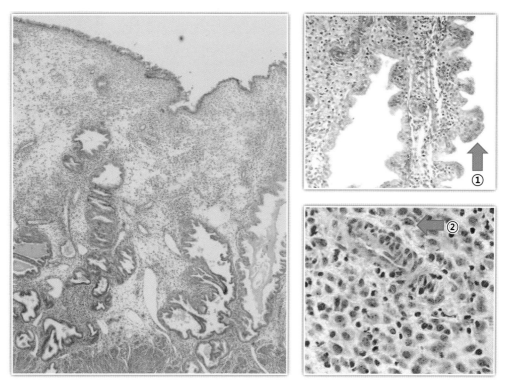

① The serrated appearance of the coiled glands
② Stromal predecidual reaction

06 Arias-Stella reaction

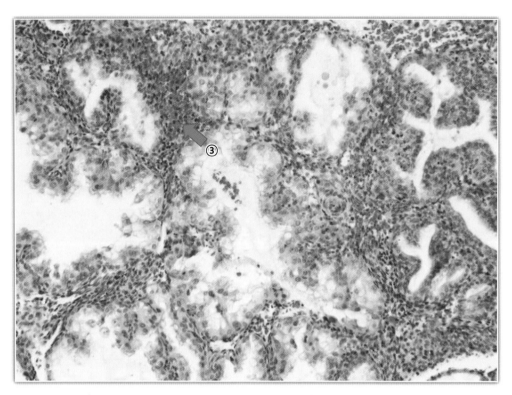

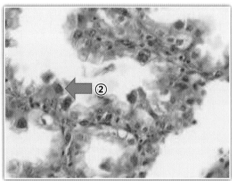

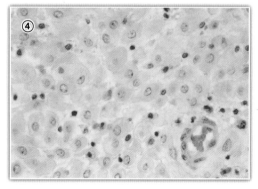

① Pregnancy, abortion, ectopic pregnancy, trophoblastic disease시 endometrial gland에서 보임

② Nuclear pleomorphism & hyperplastic glandular change

③ Stroma가 사이사이 관찰됨

④ Stromal decidualization

II. Infection of endometrium

01 Pyometra

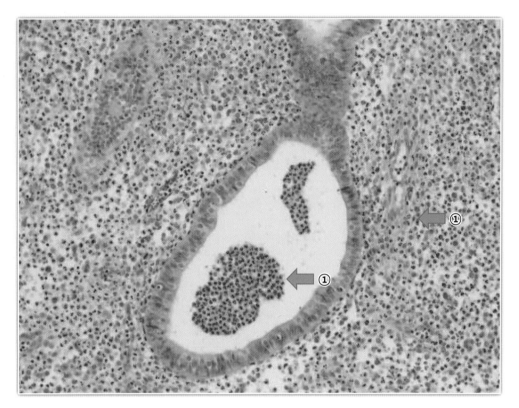

① Accumulation of pus in the uterine lumen

② Abundant neutrophils

02 Chronic endometritis

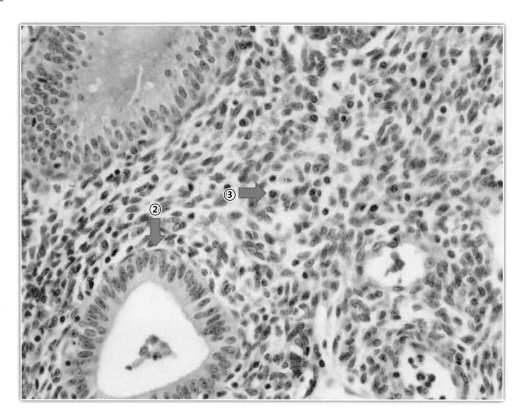

① Spindly stroma with edema : Focal early breakdown with surface neutrophils

② Associated with weakly proliferative glands

③ Plasma cells(한쪽으로 치우친 핵, purple color)

④ Focal necrosis or focal calcification

03 Tuberculosis

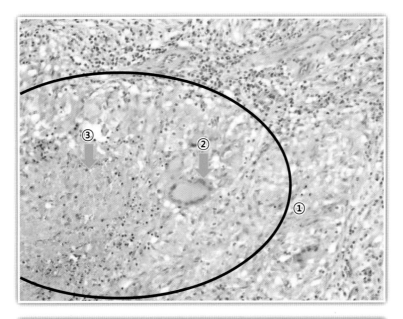

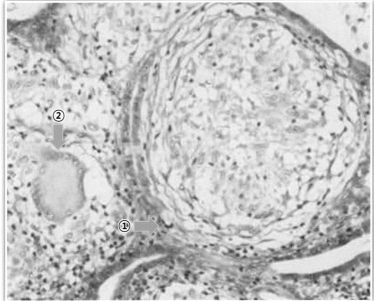

① Granulomas tend to accumulate in superficial functional layers of endometrium

② Multinucleated giant cells in granuloma

③ Necrosis

III. Abnormal uterine bleeding & pain of endometrium

01 Abortion

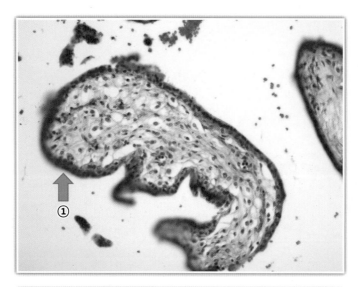

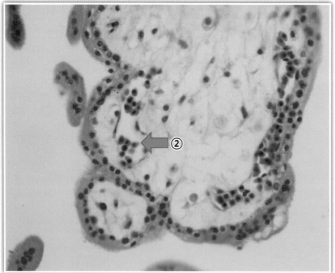

① Chorionic villi

② Fetal RBCs

③ Syncytiotrophoblasts and Cytotrophoblasts

02 Endometrial polyp

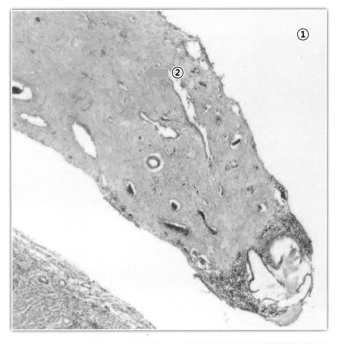

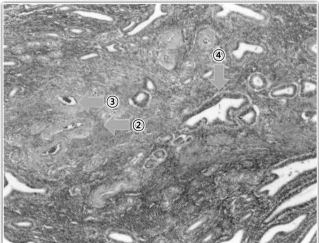

① Polypoid shape

② Fibrotic stroma

③ Thick-walled feeding vessels

④ Glands are proliferative or inactive but usually peripheral and are typically angulated

03 Adenomyosis

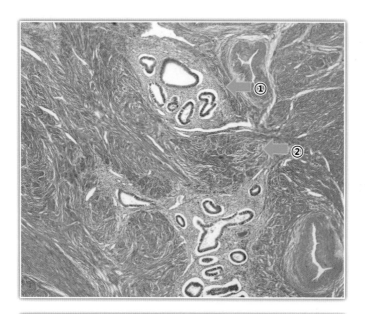

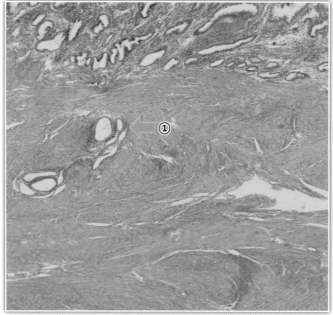

① Stroma plus marker glands deep in myometrium

② Often smooth muscle hypertrophy present around glands

③ Usually consists of basal layer of endometrium that may be connected with mucosa

IV. Precursors of epithelial tumors of the endometrium

01 Simple hyperplasia without atypia

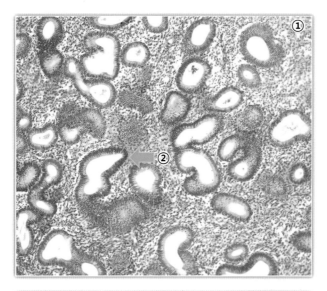

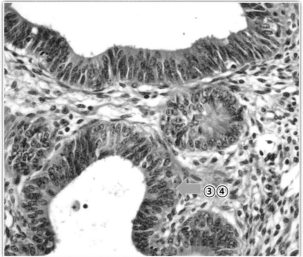

① Stroma에 비해 gland의 비율이 1:1 이상

② Glands usually round, but may be irregular with cystic dilation

③ Lining epithelium is pseudostratified or mildly stratified

④ Without atypia : 진하면서 키가 큰 길쭉한 핵으로 구성

02 Complex hyperplasia without atypia

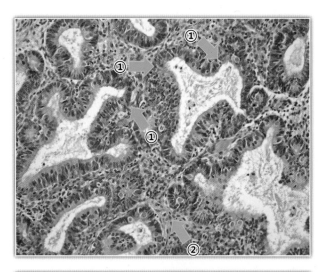

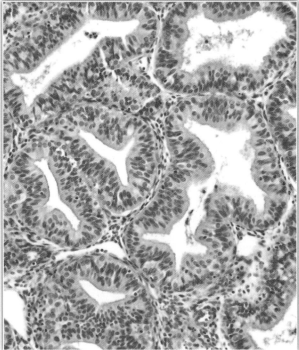

① Increase in number and size of endometrial glands with crowding of stroma and budding

② Some normal stromal cells are present between adjacent glands

③ Complex pattern may be secretory with eosinophilic metaplasia

03 Complex hyperplasia with atypia

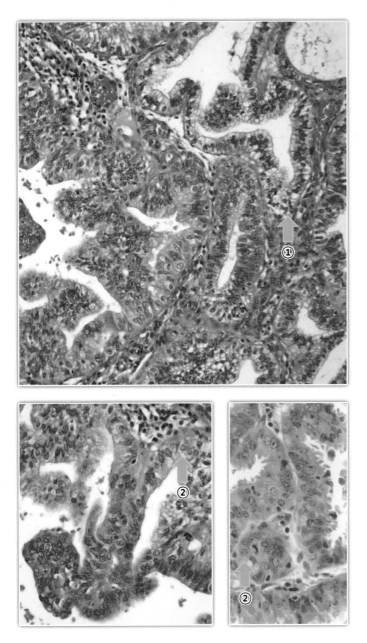

① Gland architecture : Complex hyperplasia

② Rounding of nuclei and formation of nucleoli : stratification, scalloping, tufting, loss of polarity, cytomegaly, hyperchromatism, pleomorphism and mitotic figures

V. Endometrial carcinoma

	Endometrial carcinoma Type I	Endometrial carcinoma Type II
Age	55~65 years	65~75 years
Clinical setting	Unopposedestrogen, Obesity, Hypertension, DM	Atrophy, Thin physique
Morphology	Endometrioid, Mucinous	Serous, Clear cell, Mixed mullerian tumor
Precursor	Hyperplasia	EIC
Behavior & Spread	Indolent, Lymphatic	Aggressive, Lymphatic & intraperitoneal

01 Endometrioid carcinoma

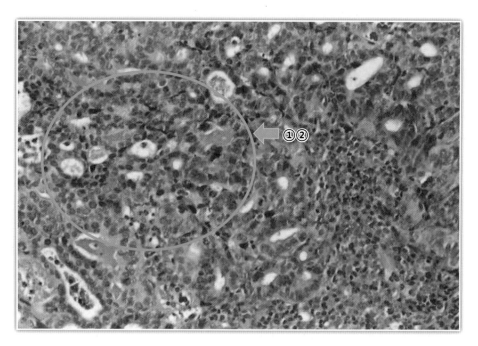

① Back to back endometrial-type glands of varying differentiation/atypia with no intervening stroma

② Cribriform glands : Fusion of glands, multiple lumens

③ Stroma present is usually desmoplastic, may have foamy cells due to tumor necrosis

④ Commonly has squamous metaplasia

02 Endometrioid adenocarcinoma

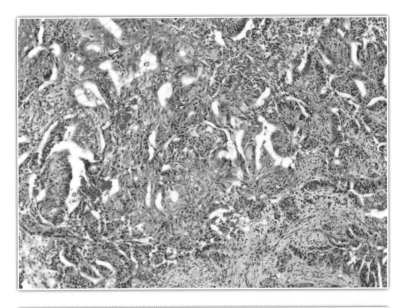

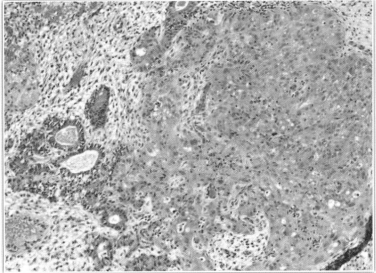

① Atypical glandular proliferation composed of tubular glands lined by columnar cells with moderate amount of eosinophilic cytoplasm and occasional intracytoplasmic mucin

② Nuclei are oval to elongated, large and stratified or pseudostratified

③ Glands can show microcysts and numerous neutrophils within and around cysts, microglandular pattern

④ Grades : vary from well differentiated to moderately to poorly differentiated

03 Endometrioid carcinoma with squamous differentiation

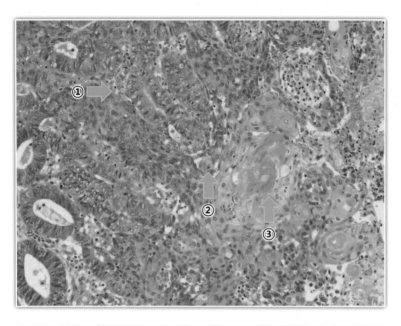

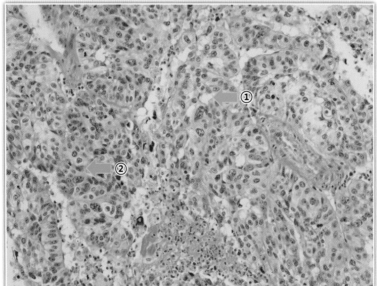

① Endometrioid carcinoma

② Squamous differentiation

③ Keratin formation

04 Endometrioid carcinoma with villoglandular pattern

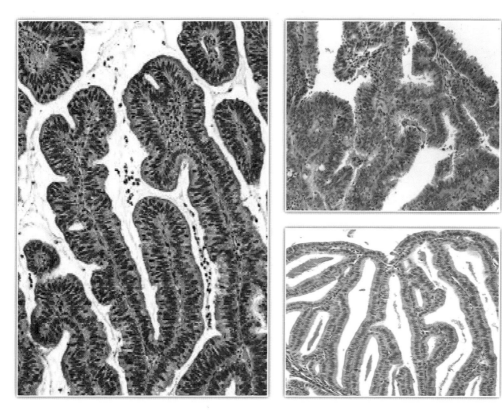

① Endometrioid carcinoma

② Well differentiated

③ Extensive, complex epithelial growth pattern with little intervening stroma

④ Villoglandular on low power

05 Serous carcinoma

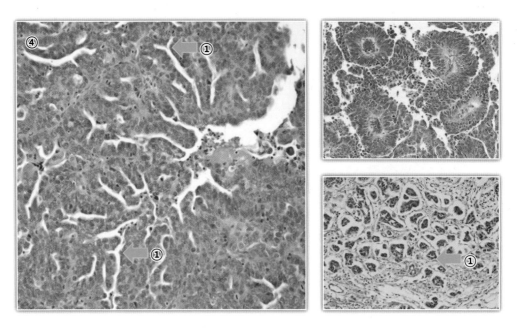

① Well-formed papillae(thick and thin) or tubules with "lobster claw" appearance containing highly pleomorphic tumor cells containing prominent nucleoli, small detached buds and tufts

② Prominent myometrial invasion, frequent mitotic activity and necrosis

③ May have glandular pattern and resemble villoglandular carcinoma

06   Clear cell carcinoma

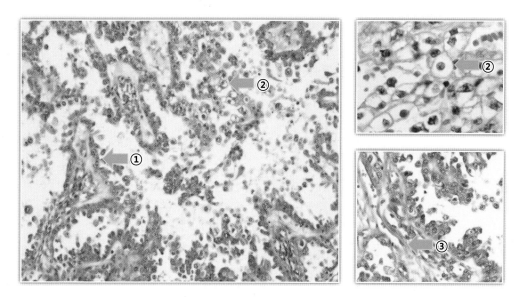

① Papillary, tubular, tubulocystic or sheet-like architecture

② Large, clear to rarely eosinophilic cells with glycogen, distinct margins and hobnail cells

③ Fibrotic stroma

④ Enlarged angulated nuclei with enlarged irregular nucleoli

VI. Smooth muscle tumors

01 Leiomyoma

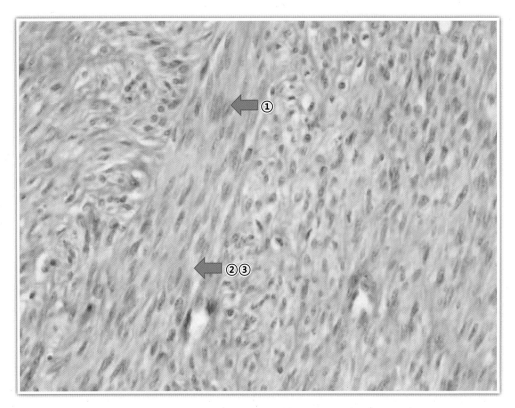

① Smooth muscle cells with bland, uniform, cigar-shaped nuclei, arranged in interlacing bundles

② Fascicular pattern of smooth muscle bundles separated by well vascularized connective tissue

③ Smooth muscle cells are elongated with eosinophilic or occasional fibrillar cytoplasm and distinct cell membranes

02 Atypical leiomyoma

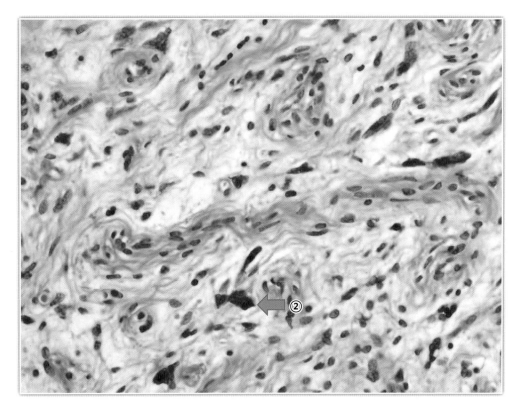

① Leiomyoma

② Atypical cell

03 Leiomyosarcoma

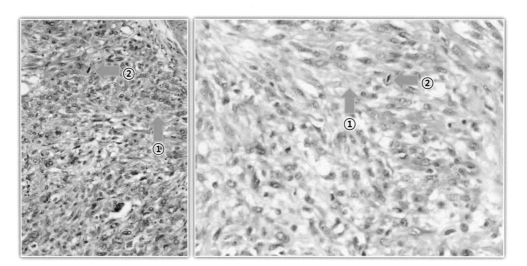

① Hypercellular

② Cellular pleomorphism & mitosis

③ Nuclear atypia

④ Tumor cell necrosis

⑤ Infiltrative/permeative

VII. Endometrial stromal tumor

01 Endometrial stromal sarcoma, low grade

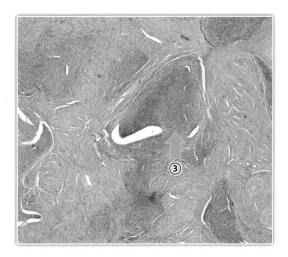

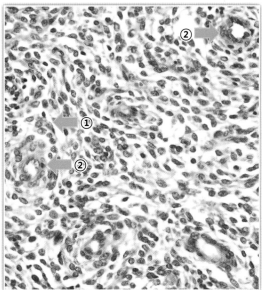

① Cytologicallybland ovoid cells proliferate in a plexiformpattern

② Prominent arterioles

③ Tongue-like infiltration between muscle bundles of myometrium

④ Angiolymphatic invasion common

VIII. Mixed epithelial and mesenchymal tumors

	Benign epithelium	Malignant epithelium
Benign mesenchyme	Adenofibroma, Adenomyoma	
Malignant mesenchyme	Adenosarcoma	Carcinosarcoma

01 Adenosarcoma

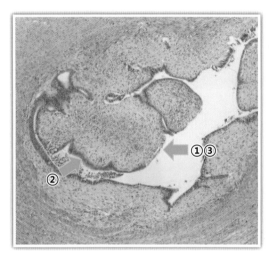
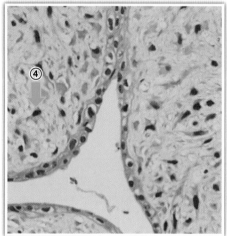

① Epithelial and stromal elements with stromal hypercellularity

② Epithelial component appears benign

③ Cystic spaces with papillary projections set in a prominent stroma

④ Variable mitotic activity in stroma

02 Carcinosarcoma (Malignant Mixed Mullerian Tumor, homologous type)

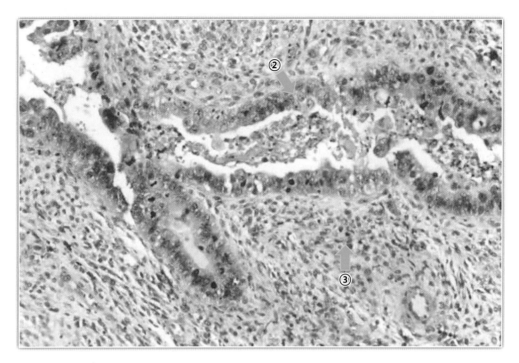

① Biphasic tumor with carcinomatous and sarcoma-like elements

② Most common epithelial component is glandular(endometrioid, clear cell, serous) and usually poorly differentiated

③ Most common sarcomatous components are homologous(endometrial stromal sarcoma, leiomyosarcoma)

03 Carcinosarcoma (Malignant Mixed Mullerian Tumor, heterologous type)

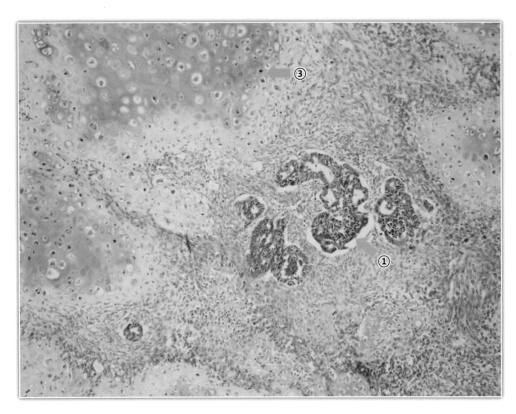

① Biphasic tumor with carcinomatous and sarcoma-like elements

② Most common epithelial component is glandular(endometrioid, clear cell, serous) and usually poorly differentiated

③ Most common sarcomatous components are heterologous(muscle, cartilage, osteoid, fat)

04 Adenomatoid mesothelioma

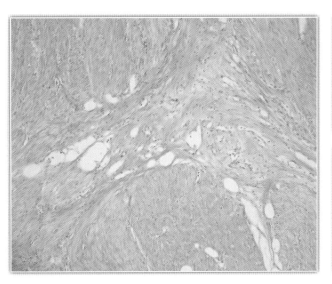
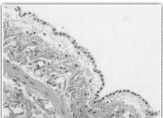
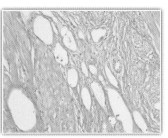

① Usually tubular spaces of varying size composed of flattened cells resembling endothelium

② Rarely large cells with eosinophilic cytoplasm

③ Often with smooth muscle hyperplasia, lymphocytic follicles

④ May have cytoplasmic vacuoles, infiltrative-like borders, clusters or small cords of cells

⑤ Rare mitotic figures, minimal atypia

I. Serous tumors

01 Serous cystadenoma

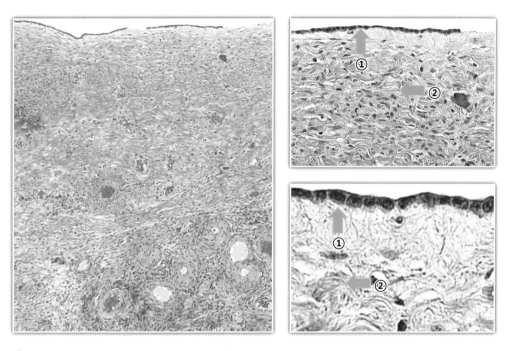

① Usually small, uni- to multi-locular cysts lined by a single layer of tall, columnar, ciliated cells resembling normal tubal epithelium or cuboidal non-ciliated epithelium resembling ovarian surface epithelium

② Stroma contains spindly fibroblasts

③ If papillae are present, they are simple papillary processes

④ No atypia, no architectural complexity, no invasion

02 Serous cystadenofibroma

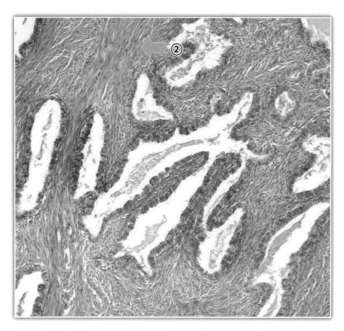

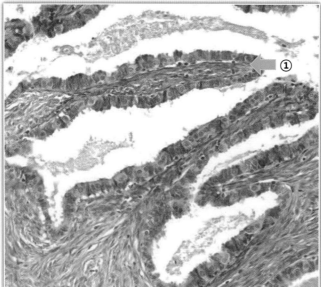

① Resemble serous cystadenoma

② Dense, fibrous connective tissue with interspersed glandular spaces

③ More pronounced proliferation of fibrous stroma

03 Serous borderline tumors

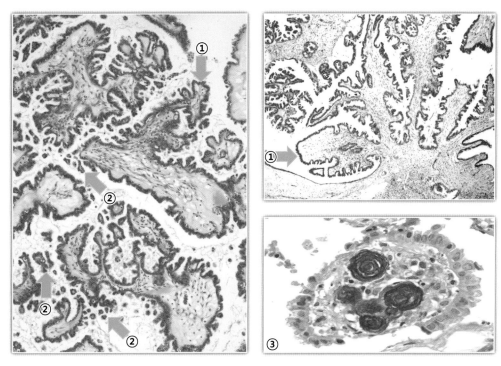

① Broad, branching papillae(hierarchical branching) focally covered by stratified epithelium with mild to moderate atypia with few mitoses

② Proliferation, tufting

③ Stroma is fibrous and edematous with variable psammoma bodies

④ Absence of destructive stromal invasion

04 Serous borderline tumors, micropapillary pattern

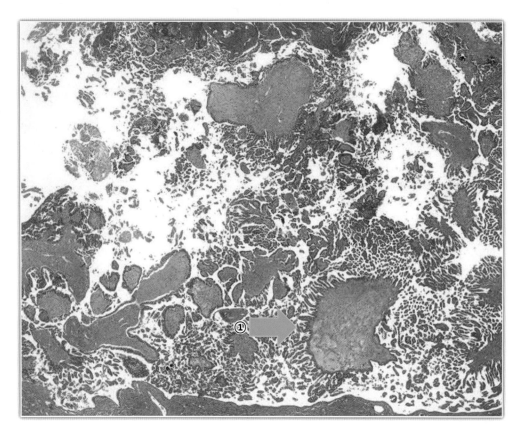

① Epithelial cells surround prominent, nonbranching fibrous stalk and protrude radially as long, thin micropapillae without cores (Medusa head)

② Marked epithelial cell proliferation

③ Only mild nuclear atypia (G1)

④ More common bilateral, exophytic, and advanced stage than typical serous borderline tumors

05 Low grade serous adenocarcinoma (LGSC)

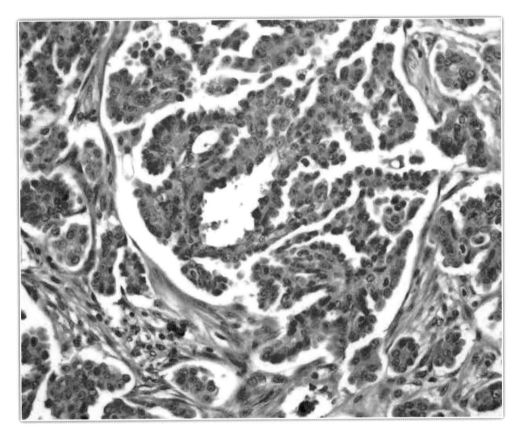

① Extensively papillary with many psammoma bodies

② May have papillae, glands, cribriform glands, cysts, or irregular nests of cells with uniform round to oval nuclei with evenly distributed chromatin, variable nucleolus

③ Mitotic index <12 MI/10HPF (secondary feature)

06 High grade serous adenocarcinoma (HGSC)

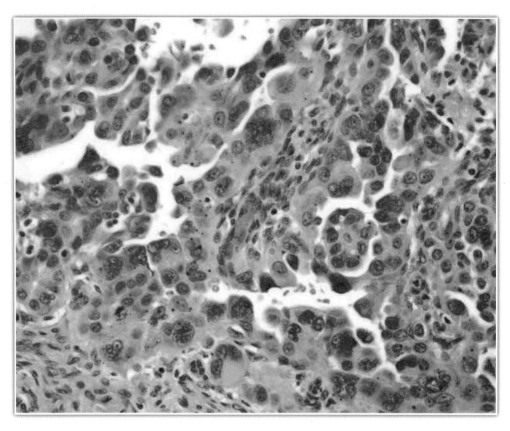

① Branching papillary fronds, slit-like fenestrations, glandular complexity, moderate to marked nuclear atypia with marked pleomorphism, prominent nucleoli, stratification, frequent mitoses, stromal invasion

② Variable psammoma bodies

③ Stroma may be fibrous, edematous, myxoid, or desmoplastic

④ Mitotic index >12 MI/10HPF (secondary feature)

II. Mucinous tumors

01 Benign mucinous tumors

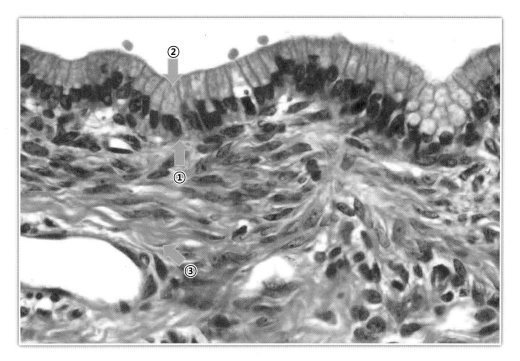

① Tall, columnar, nonciliated cells, basal nuclei

② Abundant intracellular mucin

③ Stroma may be fibrous or mimic ovarian stroma

02   Mucinous borderline tumors, intestinal type

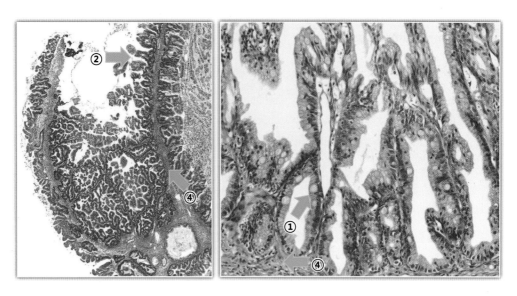

① Resemble dysplastic intestinal epithelium with goblet cells, neuroendocrine cells

② Neoplastic cells have hyperchromasia, crowding, increased mitosis, stratification forming papillae with thin fibrous cores

③ ≥10 % : Atypical epithelial proliferation without stromal invasion

④ No stromal invasion

03 Mucinous borderline tumors, endocervical type

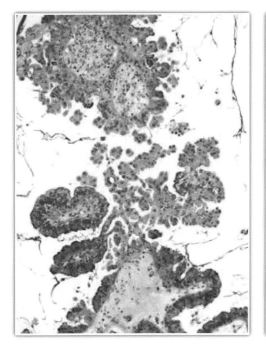 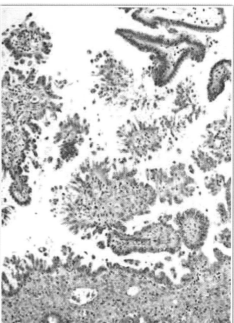

① Contain broad papillae lined by benign appearing stratified mucinous and eosinophilic endocervical-
like cells

② Brisk neutrophilic response

③ Intraepithelial carcinoma and microinvasion are rare

04 Mucinous cystadenocarcinoma, expansile type

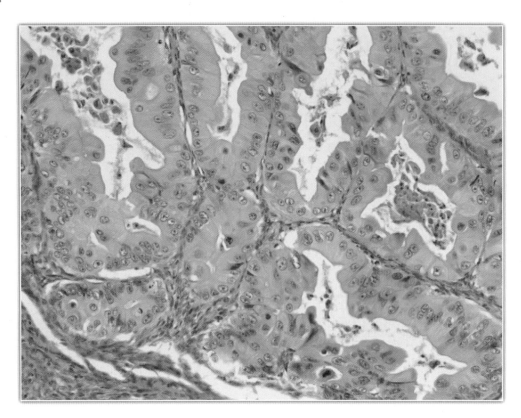

① Unilateral & Size >10 cm

② Smooth external surface

③ Complex papillary pattern

④ Microscopic cystic glands, necrotic luminal debris, mural nodules

⑤ No destructive stromal invasion

05 Mucinous cystadenocarcinoma, infiltrative type

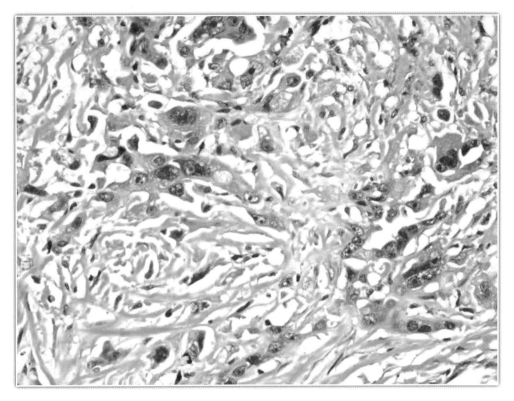

① Resemble expansile type

② Destructive stromal invasion

06 Pseudomyxoma peritonei

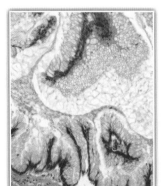
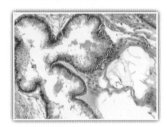
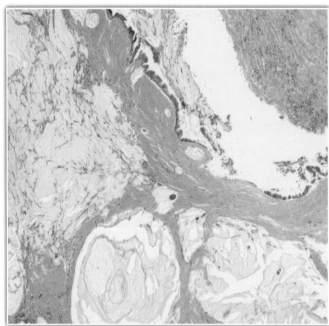

① Primary site : Appendix

② Abundant gelatinous pelvic/abdominal mucin or mucinous ascites accompanied by peritoneal lesions with bland to low-grade adenomatous mucinous epithelium intimately associated with pools of extracellular mucin and fibrosis

③ Peritoneal mucinous tumor/ascites almost always has mucinous epithelium present

III. Endometrioid tumors

01 Endometriosis

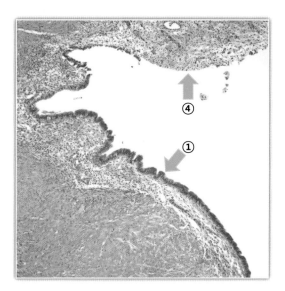

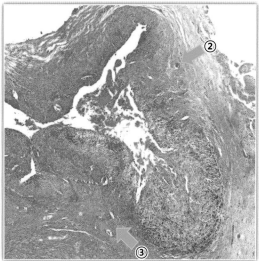

① Needs 2 of 3 features of endometrial glands, endometrial stroma or hemorrhage

② Stromal cells have naked nuclei and are surrounded by reticulin and spiral arterioles

③ Smooth muscle stroma is common

④ Repeated hemorrhage may destroy stromal tissue

02 Endometrioid adenofibroma

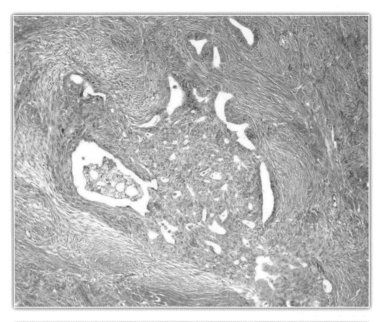

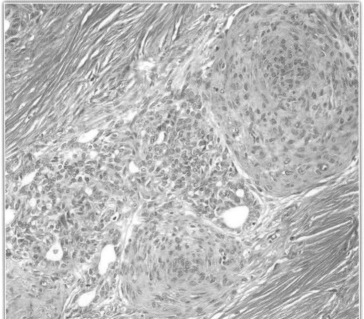

① Endometroid and fibroma-like features

② There should be no cytologic or architectural atypia

03   Endometrioid borderline tumor

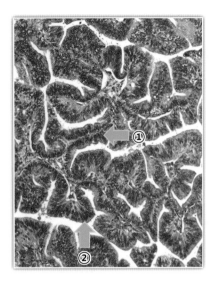 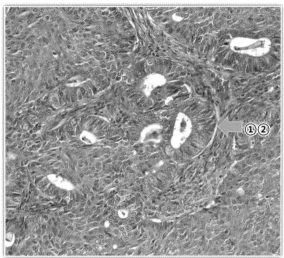

① Composed of aggregates, glands or cysts of endometrioid-type epithelium that is atypical or cytologically malignant

② May have architectural atypia including non-branching villous papillae, cribriform glands but lacks destructive stromal invasion, glandular confluence or stromal disappearance

③ Often has adenofibromatous pattern(47%) or squamous differentiation(47%)

04 Endometrioid adenocarcinoma

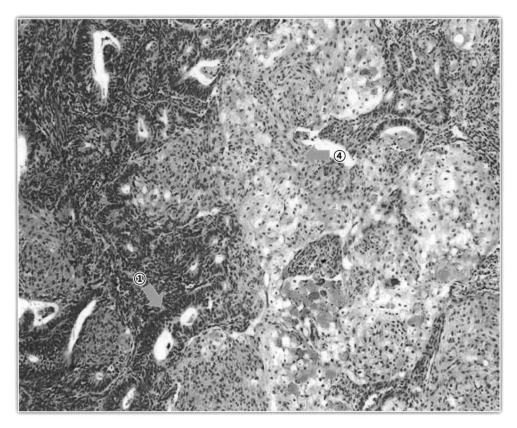

① Either non-cystic villoglandular pattern, glandular confluence or stromal disappearance

② Stromal invasion is defined as confluent glandular growth, stromal disappearance or obvious stromal invasion

③ Resembles endometrioid adenocarcinoma of endometrium, usually well differentiated

④ 50% have squamous metaplasia(morules or keratin pearls, formerly called adenoacanthomas)

IV. Clear cell tumors

01 Clear cell carcinoma

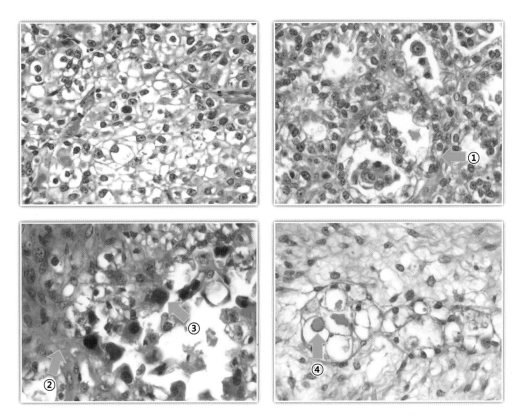

① Tubular-cystic, papillary or solid

② Papillary cores have prominent hyalinization

③ Large tumor cells, some with nuclei that protrude into lumina(hobnail cell)

④ Large tumor cells, some with clear cytoplasm(glycogen, mucin, fat)

V. Brenner tumors

01 Brenner tumor, benign

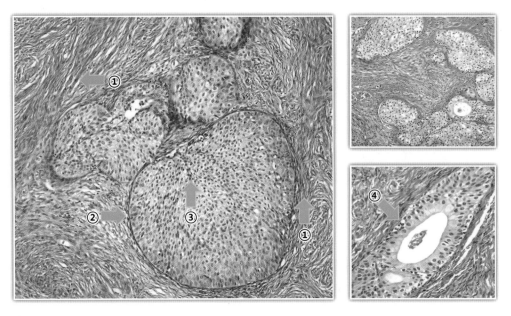

① Solid and cystic nests of urothelium-like cells surrounded by abundant dense, fibrous stroma

② Epithelial cells have sharp outlines

③ Cells are uniform, polygonal with pale cytoplasm, small but distinct nucleoli, often grooved nuclei
(similar to granulosa cell tumors)

④ Frequent microcysts within epithelial nests

02 Brenner tumor, borderline

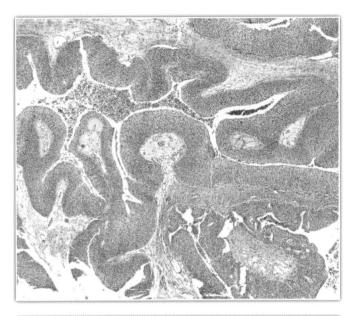

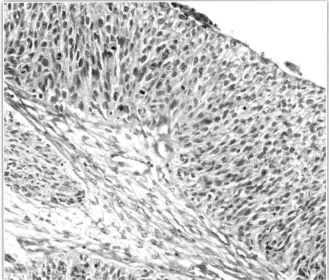

① Solid and papillary epithelial proliferation with moderate to high grade nuclear atypia

② Papillary areas lined by multilayer epithelium

③ Cells have prominent nucleoli, nuclear grooves

④ No stromal invasion

03 Brenner tumor, malignant

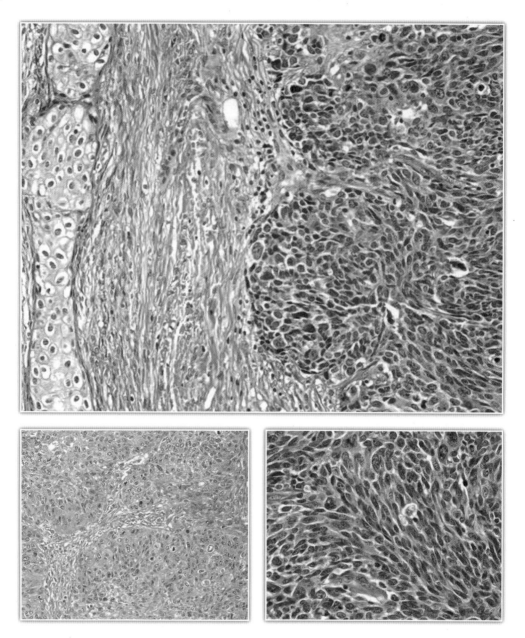

① Resembles urothelial, squamous or undifferentiated carcinoma, but associated with benign or borderline Brenner component

② Stromal invasion is present

VI. Pure stromal tumors

01 Fibroma

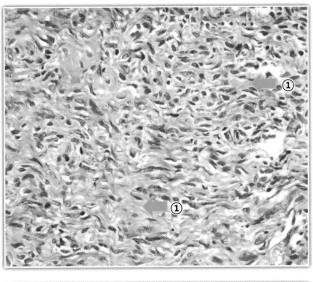

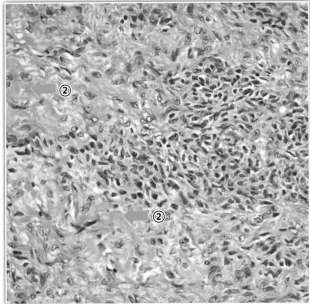

① Closely packed spindle cells in "feather-stitched" or storiform pattern

② May have hyaline bands and edema, no atypia

02 Cellular fibroma

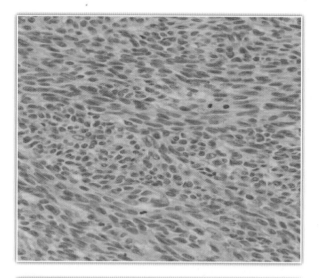

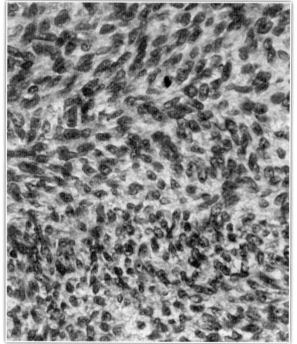

① Densely cellular with scanty collagen

② Mild atypia

③ Mitosis <3/10HPF

03 Thecoma

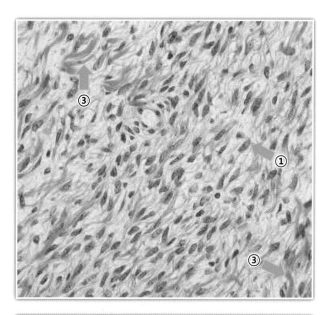

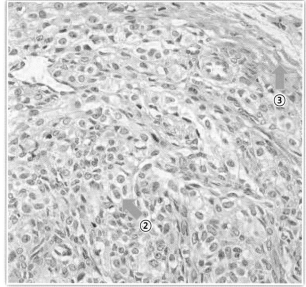

① Spindle cells with moderate pale cytoplasm containing lipid droplets and central nuclei

② Sheets of uniform cells with oval to round nuclei

③ Intervening stroma has collagen deposition and focal hyaline plaque formation

④ Some tumors are heavily calcified(stromal hyperplasia, hyperthecosis)

04 Fibrothecoma

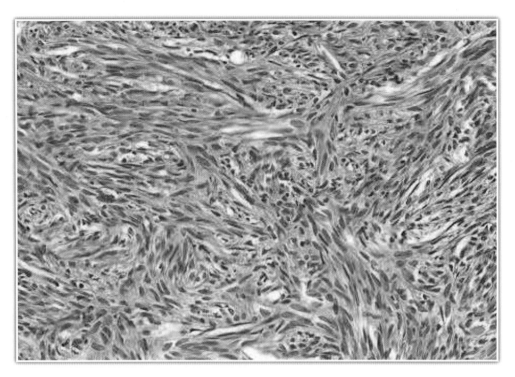

① Combined fibroma and thecoma

② Generalized term for these two closely related tumors

05 Fibrosarcoma

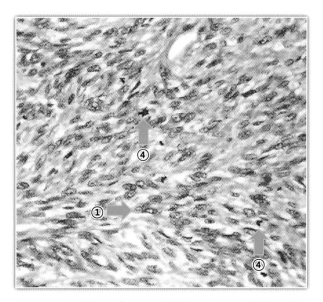

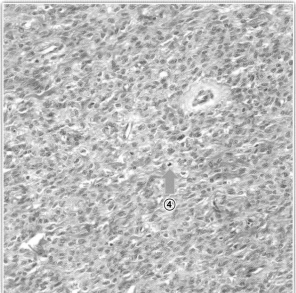

① Spindle cells arranged in sheets and intersecting fascicles creating a diffuse herringbone appearance

② Mild to moderate nuclear atypia

③ Reticulin stain separates individual neoplastic cells

④ Mitotic activity >4/10HPF : Most important criteria for diagnosing fibrosarcoma

VII. Pure sex-cord tumors

01 Adult granulosa cell tumor

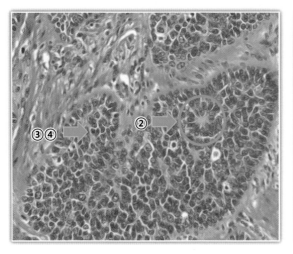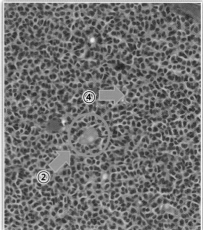

① Small, bland, cuboidal to polygonal cells in various patterns

② Call-Exner bodies : Small fluid-filled spaces between granulosal cells in ovarian follicles and in ovarian tumors of granulosal origin

③ Cells have coffee bean nuclei with folds/grooves

④ Central round nuclei with single prominent nucleoli

02 Juvenile granulosa cell tumor

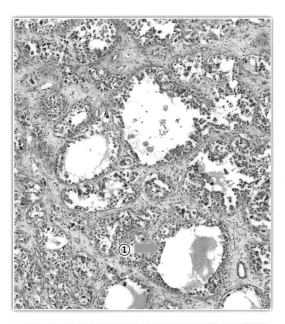

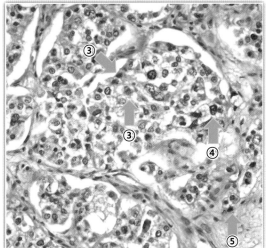

① Round to oval follicle

② Mucinous secretion

③ Luteinized granulosa & theca cells

④ Hyperchromatic nuclei

⑤ Mitosis, atypical mitosis

03 Sertoli-Leydig cell tumor, well differentiated

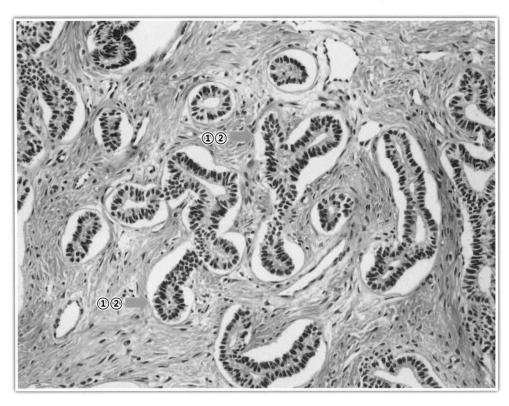

① May be nodular : Tubular (hollow > solid)

② Easily identifiable Leydig cells and Sertoli cells in a tubular pattern : May resemble endometrioid
carcinoma or atrophic seminiferous tubules

04 Sertoli-Leydig cell tumor, intermediate differentiation

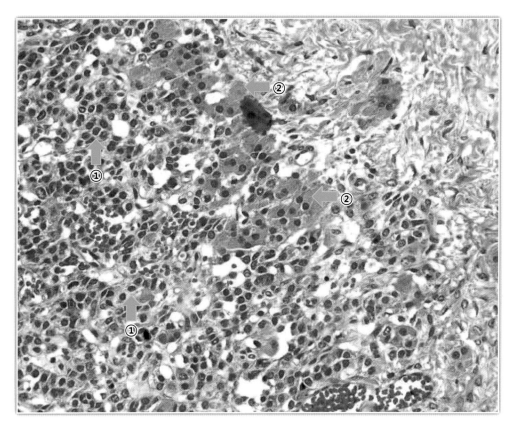

① Ill-defined mass of immature Sertoli cells

② Large eosinophilic Leydig cells separated by spindle stroma

05 Sertoli-Leydig cell tumor, poorly differentiated

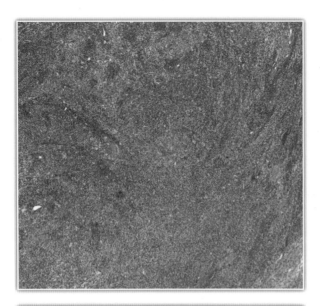

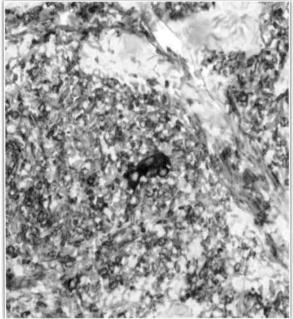

① Resemble indifferent gonad : May have sarcomatous appearance

② Leydig cells in 2/3 : May have mucus filled epithelial cells, cartilage, skeletal muscle

③ Differential diagnosis by inhibin alpha stains

VIII. Germ cell tumors

01 Dysgerminoma

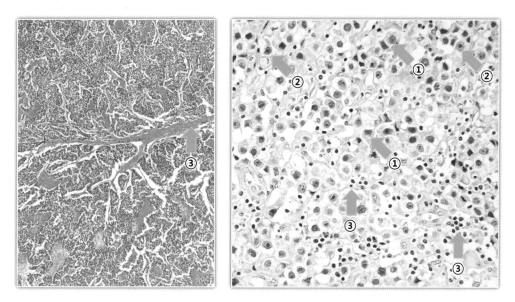

① Large round, ovoid or polygonal cells having abundant, clear, very pale-staining cytoplasm

② Large and irregular nuclei with prominent nucleoli

③ Fibrous septa with extensive infiltration of lymphocytes, plasma cells

02 Endodermal sinus tumor

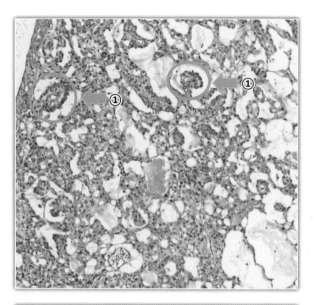

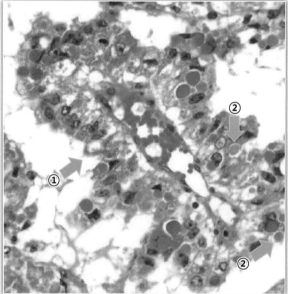

① Schiller-Duval body : Central blood vessel enveloped by germ cells within a space similarly lined by germ cells, resembles glomerulus

② Hyaline droplets present in all tumors

③ Numerous patterns

03 Mature teratoma

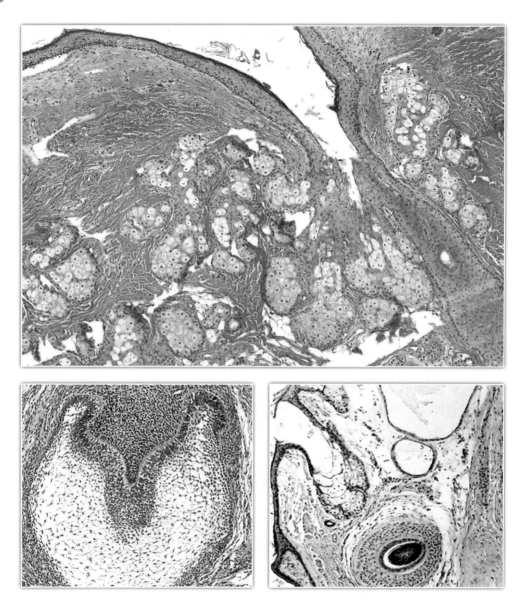

① Ectodermal structures in 100%, mesodermal in 93% and endodermal in 71%

② Skin and glial tissue common, prostate tissue in 10%

③ Still considered mature if microscopic foci of immature tissue

04 Immature teratoma

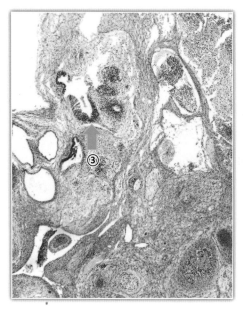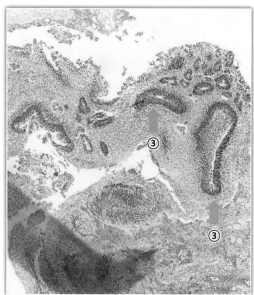

① Mixture of mature and immature elements

② Immature : Embryonal-type tissue

③ Neuroepithelial tubules & rosettes admixed with hypercelluar glia with numerous mitoses

④ Immature cartilage, bone, skeletal muscle, glands

⑤ Embryonal endodermal element : Hepatic or intestinal epithelium

IX. Metastatic carcinoma

01 Krukenberg tumor

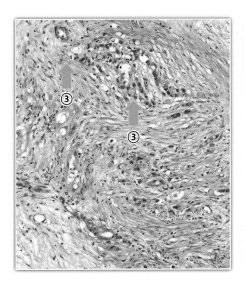 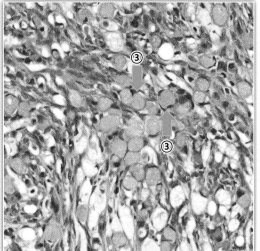

① Multiple nodules separated by normal stroma in small tumors and focally in large tumors

② More cellular at periphery and edematous, gelatinous centrally

③ Signet-ring cell : Mucin produce

④ Intracytoplasmic mucin : commonly vascular space invasion

⑤ May have marked stromal proliferation with storiform growth and variable luteinization

⑥ Frequently focal tubule, glands and cysts

02 Metastatic colon carcinoma

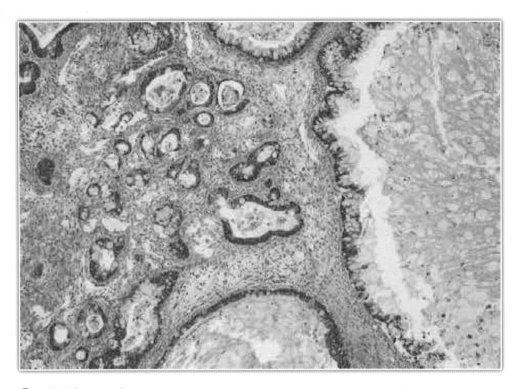

① Well differentiated

② Cribriform growth

③ Intraluminal "dirty" necrosis

④ Segmental destruction of glands

⑤ No squamous metaplasia

X. Non-neoplastic disorders

01 Tuboovarian abscess

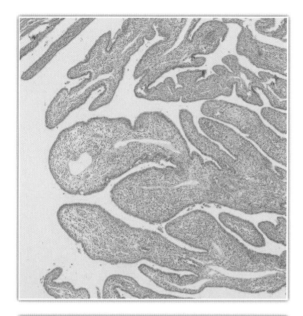

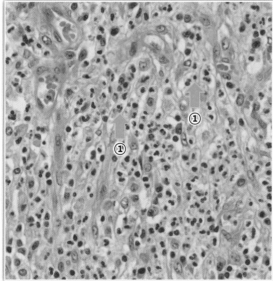

① Ovarian stroma is replaced by collagenous tissue containing numerous chronic inflammatory cells

② Cyst wall often contains ovarian stroma

02 Actinomycosis

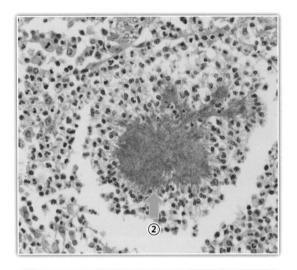

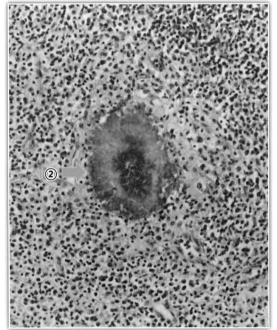

① Marked capsular fibrotic thickening with thick fibrous bands dividing nodes into nodules

② Sulfur granules : Fine filaments radiating from the periphery of the clumps

③ No palisading of histiocytes around the abscesses

④ Numerous macrophages are present in germinal centers

03 Pelvic tuberculosis

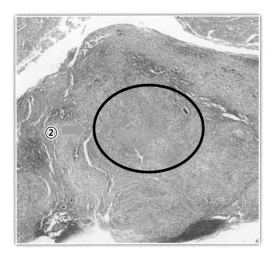

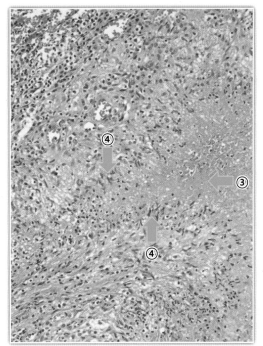

① Tuberculosis is typically confined to the cortex

② Granuloma : Caseous necrosis with epithelioid histiocytes

③ Caseous necrosis

④ Epithelioid histiocytes

XI. Tumor-like lesions

01 Multiple theca lutein cysts

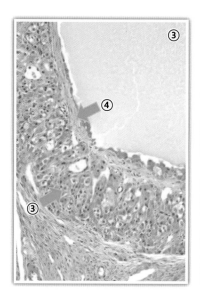 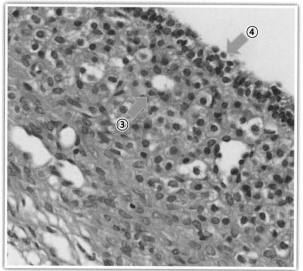

① Bilaterally enlarged ovaries with multiple theca lutein cysts

② Follicular cysts with prominent luteinized theca interna cells & luteinized granulosa cells

③ Luteinized theca interna cells

④ Luteinized granulosa cells

⑤ Edematous stroma with luteinization

02 Luteoma of pregnancy (Nodular theca-lutein hyperplasia)

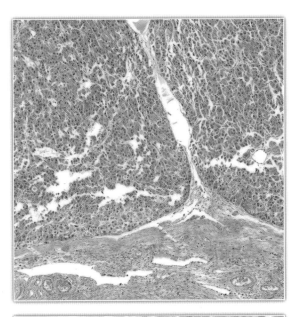

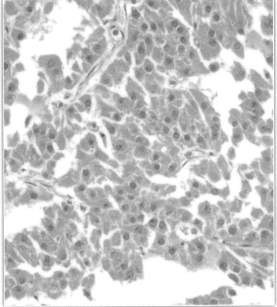

① Sharply circumscribed, rounded masses of polygonal cells with abundant pink cytoplasm containing little lipid (theca-lutein cells), round nuclei, variably prominent nucleoli, mild nuclear atypia

② 2-3 MF/10HPF, scant stroma

I. Benign squamous & glandular lesions of vagina

01 Condyloma acuminatum

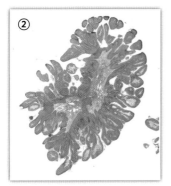

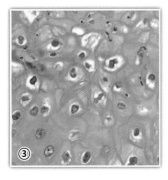

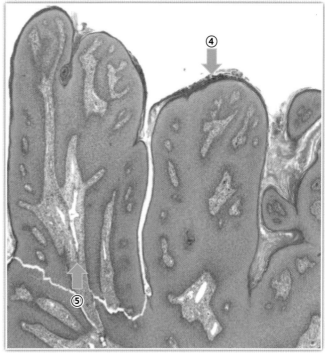

① HPV 6, 11

② Papillary growth of squamous epithelium

③ Koilocytosis : perinuclear halo & nuclear atypia

④ Hyperkeratosis

⑤ Fibrovascular core

02 Tubulosquamous polyp

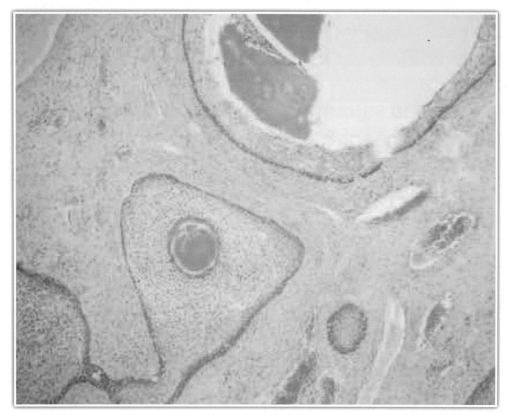

① Benign lesion composed of squamous epithelial and tubular structures set in a fibrovascular stroma

03 Fibroepithelial polyp

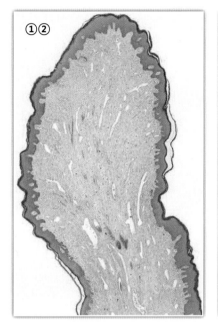 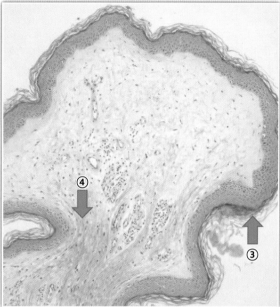

① Polypoid or pedunculate tumor-like lesion

② Papillary, fibrovascular cores covered by squamous epithelium

③ Thick epithelial surface

④ Connective tissue stalk

04 Tubovillous and Villous Adenoma

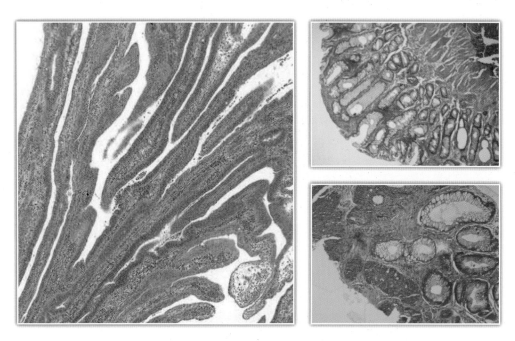

① Polyp that resemble colorectal adenoma

② Developed from intestinal, cloacal, urothelial or mullerian epithelium

II. Mesenchymal neoplasms of vagina

01 Rhabdomyosarcoma (Sarcoma botryoides)

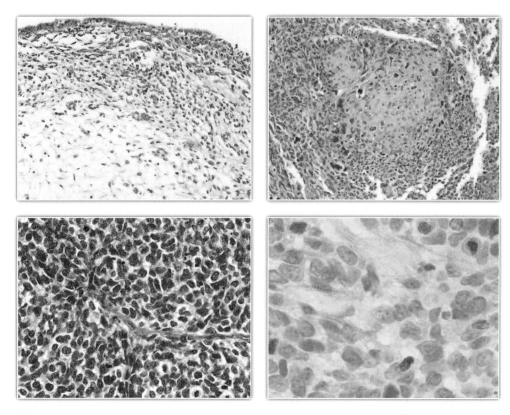

① Small tumor cells with oval nuclei, cytoplasm protrudes from one end

② Rhabdomyoblastic differentiation : Tennis rackets shape with eosinophilic granular cytoplasm

③ Tumor cells crowded into cambium layer beneath intact vaginal epithelium and around blood vessels

⑤ In deep regions, lie within loose, fibromyxoid stroma with edema and inflammatory cells

02 Adenosis

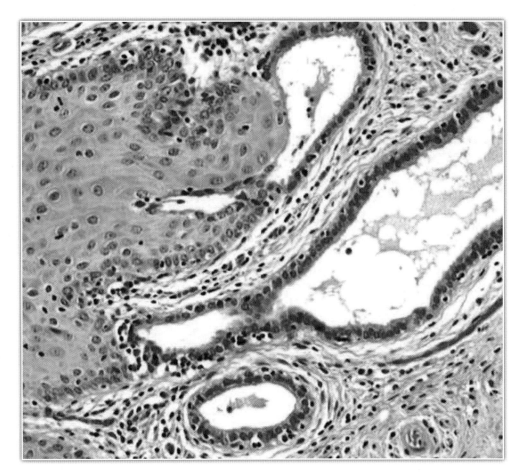

① Endocervical-type mucous glands on vaginal surface or in lamina propria, often presenting as cysts or nodules

② Tuboendometrial cells and embryonic columnar cells between lamina propria and squamous epithelium

③ Often chronic inflammation and squamous metaplasia

03   Angiomyofibroblastoma

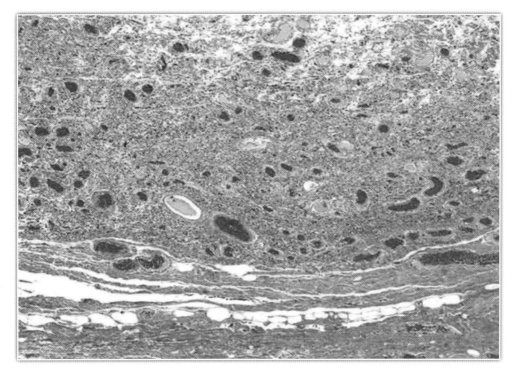

① Encapsulated tumor with hyper- and hypocellular areas and numerous vessels

② Vessels may be hyalinized

③ Hypercellular areas composed of plump stromal cells that often congregate around vessels

④ Hypocellular areas are more spindled

04 Aggressive angiomyoma

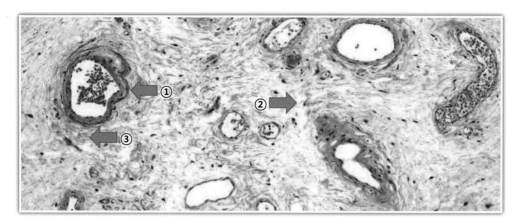

① Thin and thick walled vessels of varying caliber within a fibromyxoid stroma

② Spindled and stellate cells in hypocellular myxomatous stroma

③ Perivascular smooth muscle fibers radiating from thick-walled blood vessels

III. Benign tumor and cyst of vulva

01 Bartholin duct cyst

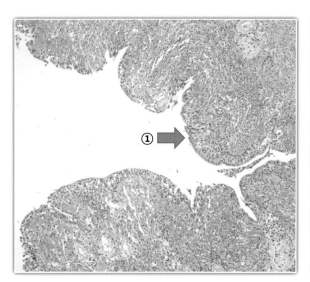 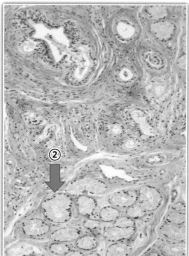

① Squamous and urothelial epithelium common, but may be destroyed by inflammatory infiltrate

② Still see residual mucinous glands with nonsulfated sialomucin

③ May have calcifications resembling malakoplakia

02 Papillary hidradenoma

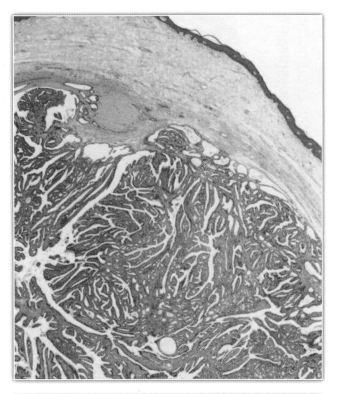

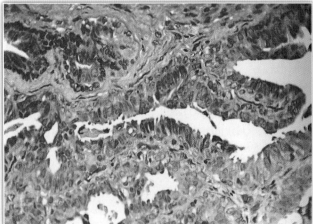

① Complicated & fine papillary growth

② Lining of epithelial cell & myoepithelial cell

③ Similarity mammary intraductal papilloma

IV. Non-neoplastic epithelial disorders of vulva

01 Lichen sclerosus

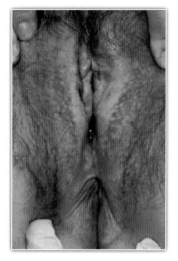 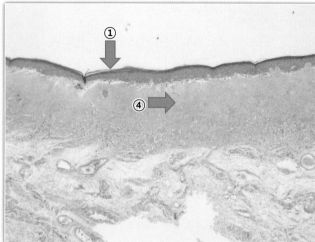

① Thinning of the epidermis

② Disappearance of rete pegs

③ Hydropic degeneration of the basal cells

④ Dermal fibrosis

⑤ Scant perivascular, mononuclear inflammatory cell infiltrate

02 Lichen simplex chronicus

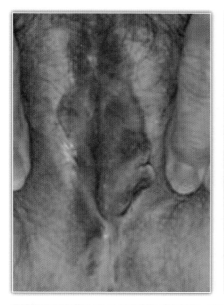
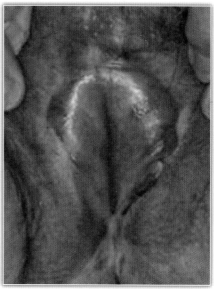

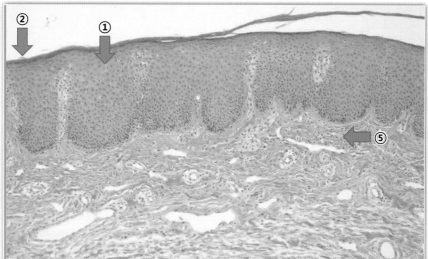

① Marked epithelial thickening

② Hyperkeratosis

③ Increased mitotic activity in basal and suprabasal layers

④ No cytological atypia

⑤ Leukocytic infiltration in the dermis

V. Epithelial tumors of vulva

01 Warty (condylomatous) type VIN

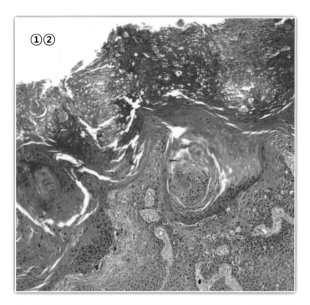

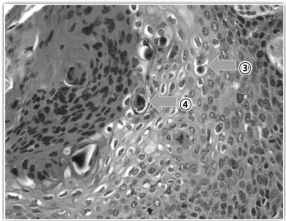

① 상피는 전형적으로 spiked surface를 보여서 "warty" 또는 "condylomatous" 모양

② 심한 상피의 증식과 parakeratosis 및 hyperkeratosis

③ 표피의 전층에서 다수의 typical 또는 atypical mitosis

④ HPV 감염 소견 : koilocytotic atypia, multinucleated cell

⑤ Atypical parakeratotic cell도 흔히 보임

02 Basaloid type VIN

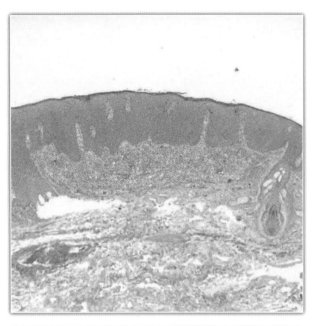

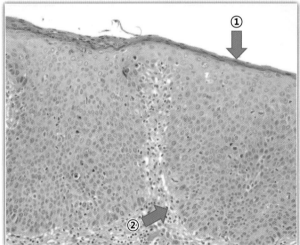

① 상피는 두꺼워져 있지만 warty VIN과는 달리 표면이 비교적 편평하고, 경도의 hyperkeratosis 와 parakeratosis가 관찰된다

② 상피는 전층이 비정형의 미성숙 parabasal type cell로 대치되어서 마치 cervix의 전형적인 in situ carcinoma와 유사한 양상을 보인다

③ 다수의 typical 또는 atypical mitosis가 관찰된다

03 Differentiated type VIN

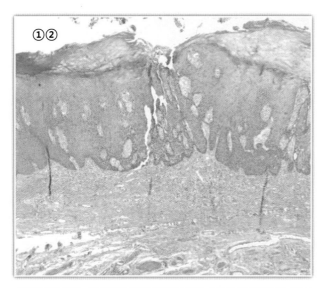

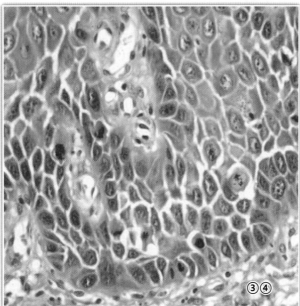

① Parabasal area에 국한된 abnormal cells

② 표층의 세포들은 정상 maturation을 보인다

③ 세포들은 prominent eosinophilic cytoplasm과 prominent nucleoli를 가짐

④ Keratin pearl

04 Paget disease

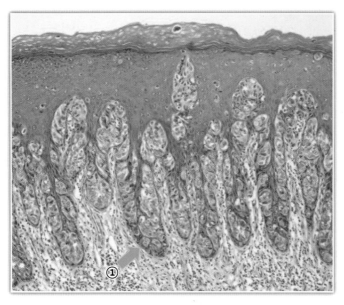

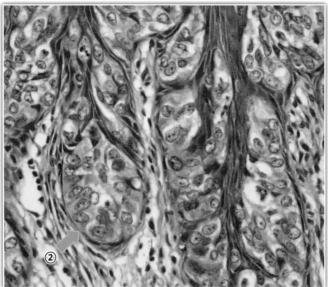

① Intraepithelial neoplasm of cutaneous origin expressing apocrine or eccrine glandular features

② Paget cells

    a. Large round cells with prominent cytoplasm (mucopolysacchride)

    b. Large nucleus and prominent nucleolus

VI. Invasive vulva cancer

01 Squamous cell carcinoma

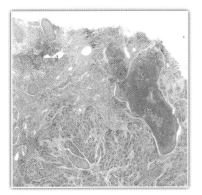 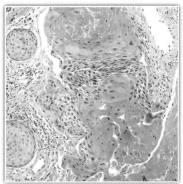

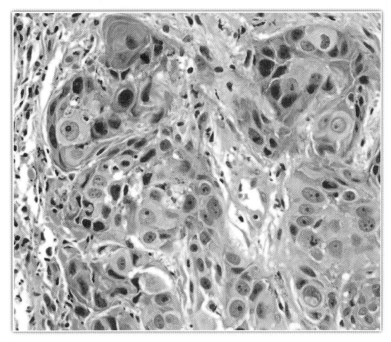

① Usually well differentiated

② Tumors on clitoris may be more anaplastic

③ VIN often present at margins

④ High grade lesions may show focal glandular differentiation, but don't call adenosquamous

02 Warty carcinoma (Condylomatous carcinoma)

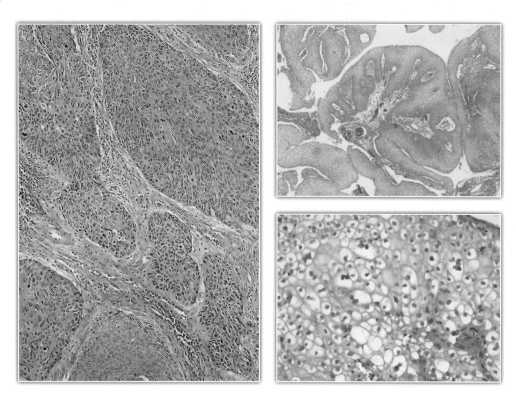

① Cellular features of HPV infection : Pleomorphism, atypia, enlargement and multinucleation, koilocytotic atypia in adjacent epithelium

② Infiltrative stromal invasion

③ Invades via single cells or clusters of cells, NOT the broad front of verrucous carcinoma

④ Associated with VIN

03 Verrucous carcinoma

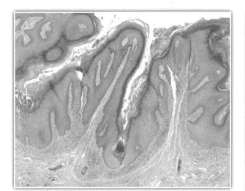
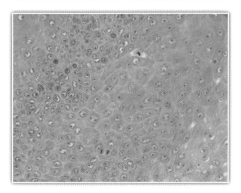
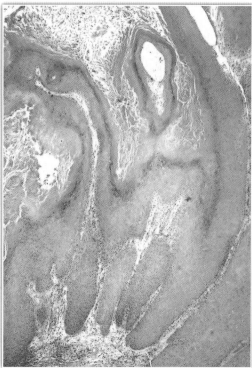

① Exo-endophytic, well circumscribed tumor composed of closely packed papillary structures lined by well differentiated stratified squamous epithelium, with minimal cellular atypia

② Epithelium demonstrates prominent acanthosis with expansion of rete ridges that push into the dermis

③ Massive hyperkeratosis and parakeratosis

④ Cells have abundant pale, eosinophilic cytoplasm with low nuclear to cytoplasmic ratio, no/mild nuclear pleomorphism

04 Malignant melanoma

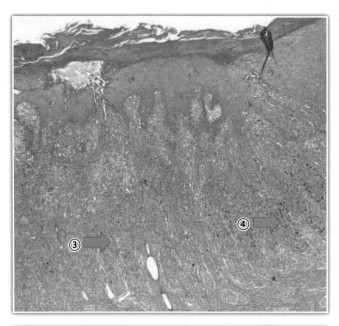

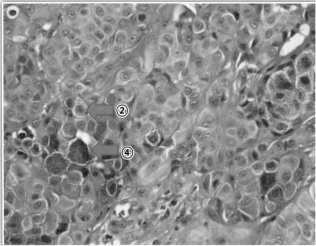

① Epithelioid or spindle cell

② Abundant eosinophilic cytoplasm, large nucleus & nucleolus

③ Radial growth phase melanomas have fibroplasia with a plaque like lymphocytic infiltrate and diffuse eosinophilic fibroplasias

④ Melanin pigment in cytoplasm

I. Disorders of Pregnancy

01 Placental membrane

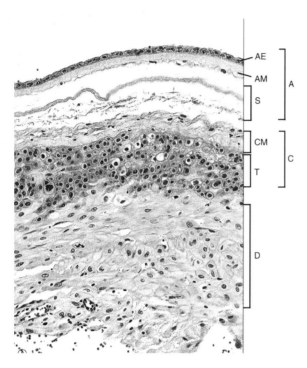

① A : Amnion

    a. AE : Amnionic epithelium

    b. AM : Amnionic mesoderm

    c. S : Spongy level

② C : Chorion

    a. CM : Chorionic mesoderm

    b. T : Trophoblast

③ D : Maternal decidua

02 Ectopic pregnancy

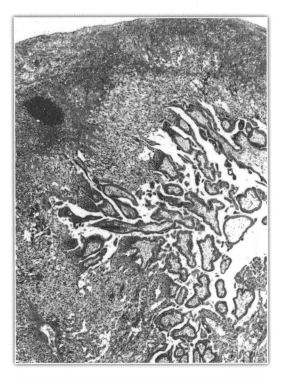

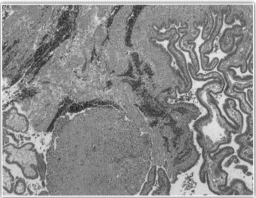

① Intraluminal chorionic villi and extravillous trophoblast(may be degenerated)

② Decidual change in lamina propria in 1/3 : Mesothelial reactive proliferation with papillary formation and psammoma bodies

③ Uterus : Gestational hyperplasia with Arias-Stella reaction, no enlarged, hyalinized spiral arteries, no fibrinoid matrix

03 Placenta accreta

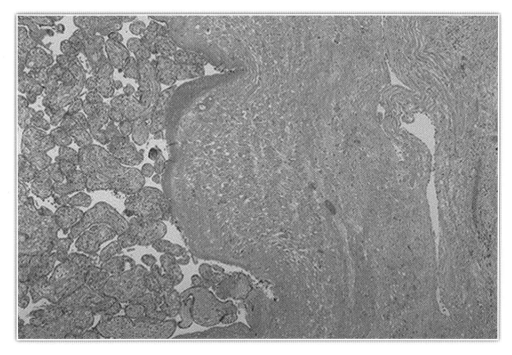

① Placental villous tissue adheres directly to the myometrium without intervening decidual plate

② Invasion of chorionic villi has occurred superficially into myometrium

04 Placental abruption

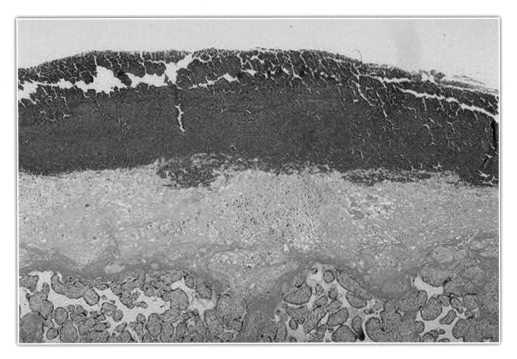

① Gross description

    a. Loose blood clots or blood clots tenuously adherent to placental floor if acute

    b. Remote episodes have brown-tan, old fibrin and necrotic tissue at abruption site and adjacent membranous tissue

    c. Features of intraplacental extension include pale areas of infarction

② Micro description

    a. Retroplacental hemorrhage or hematomas associated with diffuse intradecidual hemorrhage, villous stromal hemorrhage / edema, intervillous thrombi or infarction

    b. Chronic hemorrhage may also show hemosiderin staining

05 Chorioamnionitis

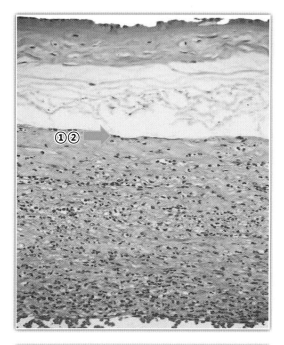

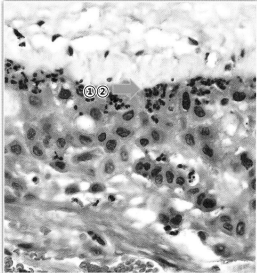

① Neutrophilic infiltrate of free membranes and those overlying the chorionic plate

② The inflammation involves the trophoblast, but not the spongy layer of the amnion

③ Variable fetal response including funisitis and chorionic plate vasculitis

06 Listeria villitis

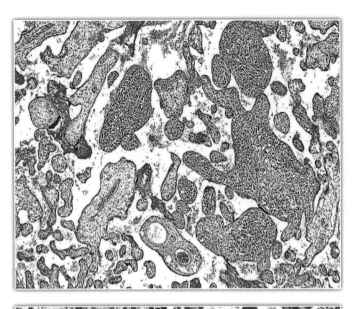

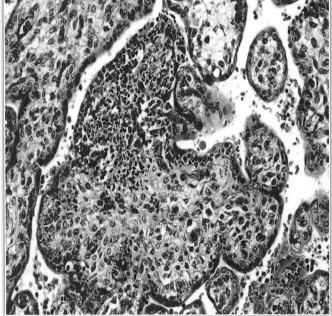

① Gram positive bacteria strongly associated with stillbirth, premature delivery and sepsis

② Acute intervillositis with intervillous microabcesses

③ Hypercellular villi

07 Cytomegalovirus (CMV)

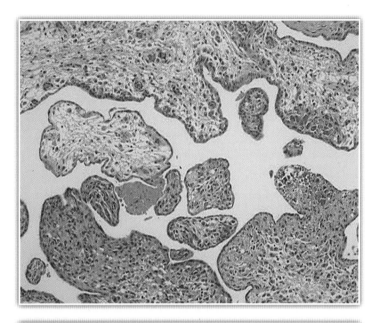

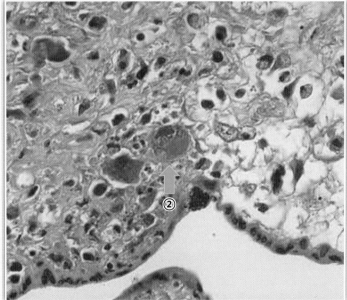

① DNA virus that causes 10% of chronic villitis cases

② Fetal CMV infection is most severe in placentas with plasmacytic villitis and inclusion bodies

③ Lymphocytic or plasmacytic villitis with hyalinized villi and mineralization

08 Acute fatty liver of pregnancy

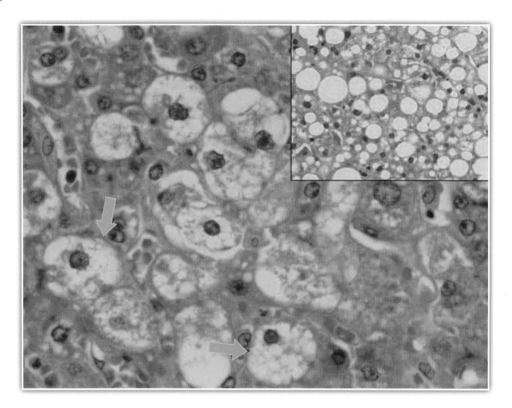

① Hepatocyte swelling

② Cytoplasm의 microvesicular fat deposition

③ Minimal hepatocellular necrosis

④ 간에만 국한되지 않고 renal tubular cell에도 lipid가 축적될 수 있음

II. Gestational Trophoblastic Disease

01 Complete hydatidiform mole

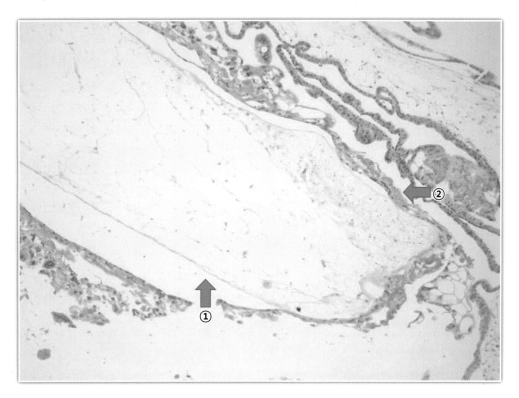

① Marked villous cavitation

② Circumferential trophoblastic hyperplasia (CT, IT, ST)

③ Cytologic atypia : 50~70%

④ No fetal component

02 Early complete hydatidiform mole

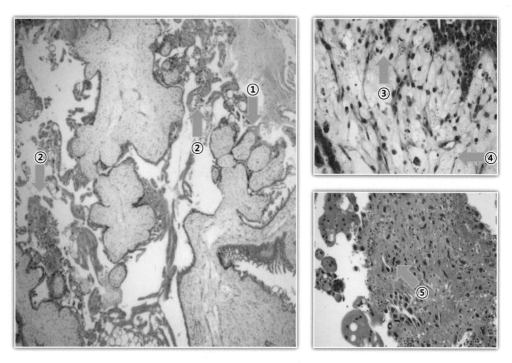

① Bulbous terminal villi reminiscent of finger knuckles

② Focal cytotrophoblast and syncytiotrophoblast proliferation

③ Myxoid stroma, sometimes cellular

④ Labyrinthine network of villous stromal canaliculi

⑤ Intermediate trophoblast atypia (nuclear and cytoplasmic enlargement, variable nuclear outlines and hyperchromasia)

03 Partial hydatidiform mole

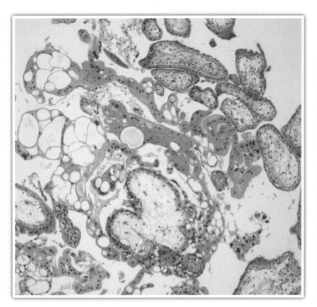 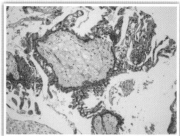 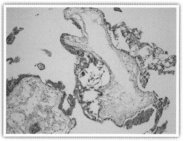

① Mixture of edematous villi similar to complete mole and relatively normal villi

② Less conspicuous central cistern formation (internal clefting)

③ Mild focal trophoblast hyperplasia without atypia

④ Villous scalloping

⑤ Villi have vessels with nucleated RBCs if fetal development present

04 Invasive mole

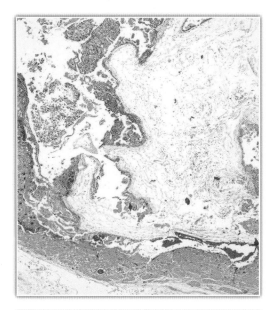

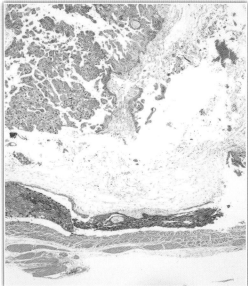

① Molar villi with trophoblast in myometrium, or extrauterine sites

② Less conspicuous hydropic villi than non-invasive mole

③ Distant metastasis : Presence of molar villi confined within blood vessel without extension into adjacent tissue

III. Trophoblastic Neoplasia

01 **Choriocarcinoma**

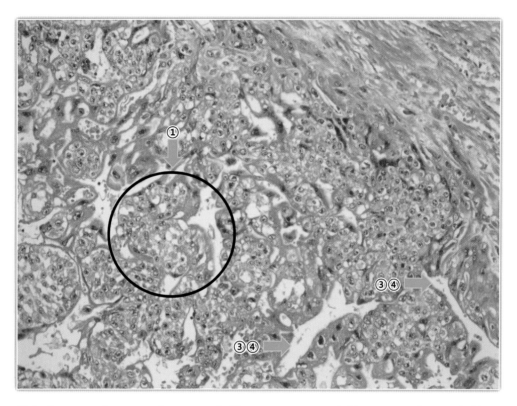

① Biphasic growth pattern : Syncytiotrophoblast capping cytotrophoblast, intermediate trophoblast

② Lack of blood vessel formation in tumor center

③ Intricate pseudovascular network & blood-lake lined by trophoblast, not endothelial cells

④ Pseudovascular channels without stromal support

⑤ Hemorrhage, necrosis and vascular invasion

02 Placental site trophoblastic tumor (PSTT)

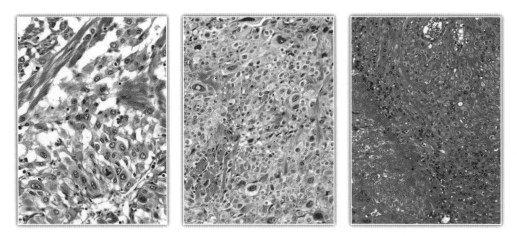

① Intermediate trophoblast proliferation that deeply invade myometrium in large nests, interdigitating pattern or masses

② No cytotrophoblast, no villi

③ Extensive deposition of fibrinoid material

④ Invasion of blood vessels with fibrinoid deposition

03 Epithelioid trophoblastic tumor (ETT)

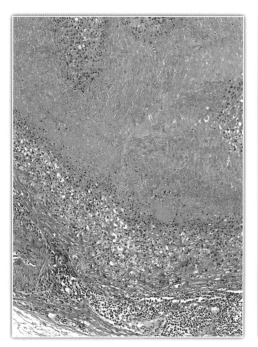 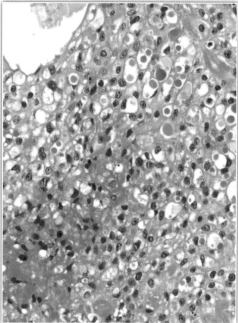

① Circumscribed tumor with pushing border

② Resembles carcinoma due to cords, nests and sheets containing hyaline material and necrotic debris

③ Mononuclear and epithelioid tumor cells resemble intermediate trophoblast of placenta

④ Have distinct cell borders, eosinophilic cytoplasm and occasional small nucleoli

⑤ Often peritumoral lymphocytic infiltrate or dystrophic calcification

04 Placental site nodule (PSN)

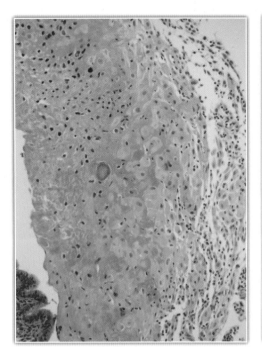 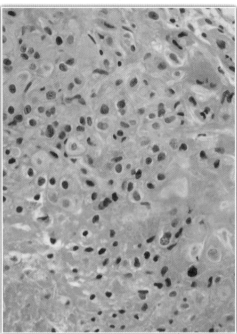

① Well-circumscribed, extensively hyalinized and paucicellular, oval or plaque like nodule

② Cells are chorionic-type intermediate trophoblast cells with abundant eosinophilic, amphophilic or clear(glycogen-rich) cytoplasm, irregular/degenerative appearing nuclei

③ Mitosis : rare or absent